MINDFULNESS FOR
BINGE EATING

By Antonia Ryan

MINDFULNESS FOR BINGE EATING

Written by Antonia Ryan.

How to Download Your Guided Meditations

To download the eight audios that accompany this book, please go to web page

www.subscribepage.com/mindfulnessaudio2.

There is a quick email registration, then you will be directed to the downloads page. You can either listen to your audios on the web, or download them to a device to use at your leisure.

When you register, you will also receive an email from me with a confirmation of the link to your downloads, which might be handy for you to refer to later. By being registered, you will have access to any updates and free resources I send out in the future. I'm sure you will want these, but you can of course unsubscribe at any time if you wish.

Downloading tips:

If you cannot access the downloads or do not receive my email with the link, the most likely reasons are:

1. There was a typo in your email address. This is easily solved by going back and resubmitting your email address again.
2. Your email service has put my email in the wrong folder. Please check folders like 'junk' and 'spam'.

If you use Gmail, it might be in the 'promotions' folder.

3. There is some sort of blocking software on your browser or device. Try using a different browser or different device.

Just in case you still have a technical problem accessing the downloads page using the method above, I have a backup system. You can also get access by sending a blank email to mindfulaudio@gmail.com. Your blank email will trigger an autoresponder that will immediately send you the access link.

Table of Contents

Introduction

Mindful eating replaces self-criticism with self-nurturing. It replaces shame with respect for your own inner wisdom.
Jan Chozen Bays.

This book is intended for anyone who struggles with overeating, binge eating, and emotional eating or food addiction issues. You may be an occasional over-eater who wishes to gain more control over their eating behaviour or on the other end of the spectrum you may have been diagnosed with Binge Eating Disorder. (B.E.D) No matter where you are on this spectrum, I hope that the guidance, advice and tips in this book will help you form a peaceful and healthy relationship with food.

If you think you are suffering from B.E.D. please get help from health care professionals. Please look on this book as an additional tool in your armoury. There is often a sense of isolation and secrecy surrounding problem eating, so reach out to support groups and talk to understanding friends.

I base my approach on mindfulness practices and much more. I will refer to a range of strategies to support you. There are many wonderful books on mindfulness, but this book is about using some of these practices in a very actionable and accessible way to help with problem eating. Although this is a very practical book I will make links with recent, relevant research. Mindfulness will only be effective if you practise it consistently so I will give you tips, hints and guidance to support you in ensuring that build these practices into your daily routine. This will maximise the impact the process will have on your eating behaviours.

I believe that a 'one size fits all' approach does not work. I will make suggestions that you can use if you feel they would help you. Some suggestions might not be right for you at the stage you are at in your recovery. What I want to do is help you trust yourself again. You are the one who will make all those micro-decisions about food, shopping, meals, snacks and eating behaviour for the rest of your life. You need to take from this book what resonates with you as an individual. You want to relax around food and trust your own judgements. I hope to offer you guidance with this.

Binge eating is a very lonely and isolating experience, shrouded in shame and secrecy. I encourage you to reach out to others, to make connections and get support. Mindfulness helps us in all our relationships; with others, with ourselves and with food.

This book will help you understand:

- Why you want to eat when you are not hungry.

- Why you have cravings for particular types of foods.

- Why you find it hard to stop eating.

- Why you judge yourself so harshly.

- Why you use food to manage emotions.

- Why food causes you so much worry and angst.

- You will discover for yourself how much food and which types of foods your body needs. You will find out which foods you really enjoy and that you can eat them without guilt or worry.

The ultimate aim of the book is to help you establish a more peaceful relationship with food, with your body and with your emotions.

I lay the book out as an eight-week program, doing just a little each day. The steps are slow, small and steady. Your disordered eating has taken a long time to develop. Healing from this will take time, effort, patience and slips. Success is never a consistent upward trajectory. However, your mindfulness practice will provide a safety net for periods when you feel you have slipped back. By being compassionate and patient with yourself, you will keep moving forward.

These steps are a long-term investment in your mental, emotional and physical health.

Finally, in this introduction, I want to acknowledge two things; first, that it takes courage to confront problem eating. I am so pleased that you have taken this step forward. Second, thank you for your trust. I aim to provide honest, responsible advice and guidance.

The Story Behind This Book.

Some years ago a friend, I shall refer to as Kim, rang me and asked if she could talk to me in confidence. Earlier that day, we had been out for coffee with a group of friends and had been chatting about our teenage years and early twenties. We got on to talking about food and how some of us had struggled, caught in a dilemma of wanting to be slim but enjoy all our favourite foods too. I had shared briefly on some issues I had with food, confidence and self-esteem in my teenage years. When I left home and had more freedom around food I had slipped into a cycle of dieting and overeating.

I had overcome these issues and Kim was keen to find out how.

Kim shared with me her own struggles with restricting food, over-exercising and binging. She shared how nervous she felt around food, always feeling that she would lose control and also about her anxieties regarding weight gain. I shared what had helped me with Kim and over the period of a few months Kim regained more trust in herself, insight into why she binged and a more relaxed attitude around food and towards her body.

This started me out on the path of helping others learn about meditation, self-acceptance and compassion and much more which I will present in this book.

About the Author.

I have worked for thirty years in the 'helping professions', teaching, supporting and coaching people of all ages and backgrounds with issues such as anxiety, stress, depression and problems with eating. I have used a variety of techniques and drawn from a range of disciplines. I have also worked in specialist units and hospital settings with people with eating disorders. In addition, I have coached people with problem eating and body image issues on a one-to-one basis. In my teens and early twenties, I struggled with these issues myself, but found peace by using the techniques outlined in this book.

This book is a synthesis of my professional and personal experience. I will refer to research to establish that my advice is not based totally on anecdotal experience but is backed up by scientific evidence.

Eating and behaviour around food is a complex, emotional and deeply personal issue. There is no 'one size fits all' diet or plan. I aim to provide a scaffolding based on mindfulness practices, I hope these practices help you as they have helped me and many people I have worked with.

Does This Sound Like You?

Maria waved goodbye to her husband and sons as they walked down the pleasant suburban street. She tried to appear relaxed and fixed a smile on her face as she waved cheerfully. She felt a stab of guilt as her two sons waved back innocently. She watched as the trio turned the corner of the street and were out of view. Maria rushed indoors and quickly pulled the curtains closed in the living room. She had told her husband that she would try to relax and watch a movie while he was out at a football match with their young sons. Maria had been looking forward to this 'me time' all week; she had tried so hard to be good. She deserved a treat. She put the television on, the only source of light in the darkened room. Maria dashed around the house and garage and gathered up the various items she had hidden.

During the week she would buy cakes, chocolate, biscuits, and ice-cream, building up the stash over time, looking forward to being on her own to indulge. Maria felt guilty about hiding these sweet treats from her children, but her compulsion to eat was too much. Maria laid out the food items with some precision and relish. She set out the ice-cream to melt a little, sat down on the floor in front of the coffee table laden with the brightly wrapped food, and pulled off the wrappers frantically, eating like someone who was ravenous.

The first few bites provided the relief Maria needed. She pushed the food in and let go of the pent up stress of the week. The stress of working full-time as a practice manager in a local doctor's surgery, of keeping the house immaculate, of worrying about her elderly father who lived two hundred miles away, each bite seemed to dull the feelings of anxiety, to loosen the grip of tension that kept her awake at night and jumpy during the day.

As Maria ate and ate, the food lost its taste, but she kept on eating more and more. The chocolate lost its sensuous appeal and tasted like wax in her mouth. Her jaws ached and her stomach felt like an over-inflated balloon. She finished the semi-liquid ice-cream, hardly registering its creamy sweetness. This was the worst bit, looking at all the wrappers and going through the routine of hiding them in the rubbish bin. Logic told her it was unlikely that her husband or sons would go through the rubbish bin, but the intense shame of them knowing what she had just done, made her face burn.

Your binge eating might look different.

Different types of binging:

- A planned binge, like Maria's.

- A slow binge over the course of an evening, lasting about four hours.

- Grazing constantly throughout the day, with no discernible mealtimes.

- Binging for comfort because you feel lonely, sad or down.

If your overeating is bothering you, this book is for you. Binge eating affects all sorts of people, including men and boys.

What binge eaters share is a pattern of eating enormous amounts of food in a short period of time with a sense of being out of control. Once you start, you can only stop when you physically cannot cram any more food into your stomach. Like Maria, binge eaters feel shame, distress, and guilt about their eating, which is usually secretive and lonely. This pattern of eating has little to do with physical hunger, is physically uncomfortable, and feels like an embarrassing secret. Binge eating seriously affects peoples' health and quality of life.

Context is highly relevant. Everyone overeats sometimes. Most people eat more than is healthy or comfortable for them at Christmas, Thanksgiving, or other festivals. This feasting is usually part of a social celebration, enjoyed with close friends and family. There is a sense of joy and pleasure in the shared food, not the intense secrecy and shame of the food crammed in during a binging session carried out in private.

Often there is anxiety about the consequences of eating so much food rich in calories and usually in sugar, fat, or salt. Some binge eaters binge on healthy food such as granola or yoghurt, but most are triggered by the heady combination of sugar, fat, salt and refined flour.

Unexpected time alone, a disappointment, or a difficult confrontation or argument might trigger a binge. Usually, food is stashed ready for this eventuality. It an emotional crutch to fall back on when life gets tough, as it will sometimes.

A binge will usually happen if there is a mix of intense, distressing or uncomfortable emotions and available highly palatable food. We talk later in the book about emotions and food addiction.

Often a binge eater can be highly motivated and disciplined in life. Binge eaters have probably followed strict diets and exercise regimes is in the past. They can hold down responsible jobs, take care of families, and are involved in the local community. They might set periods of time when they eat very little or consume only water or diet shakes to keep them going. Often this is a desperate attempt to cut down on the calories and keep the weight off.

Eating out is not usually a pleasure. Often binge eaters feel judged by others, perhaps because of their size. Although not all binge eaters live in larger bodies. They dislike eating around others and feel fearful of losing control around food. Decisions about what to order can be agonizing and feelings of being judged and ridiculed take the joy out of social occasions.

How Can Mindfulness Help?

If you are new to mindfulness, I will explain the practices. You need not know anything about mindfulness to use this book.

My understanding of mindfulness is this: that it is essentially about, keeping your attention on the present; accepting your experience of everything as it is, without pushing it away or clinging on to it.

Although mindfulness has its roots in religious traditions, mindfulness is not necessarily a religious practice. This book is a down to earth guide; you do not need any bells, candles or incense to practice mindfulness.

In this book, I will provide solutions to help you in the short term and longer-term. I will start with some strategies to help immediately, a first-aid for binge eating if you like. Although eating issues often have deep-seated causes which take time to tease out, you can get started right away. Please don't wait until you are 'fixed' to break free of overeating. You can start now, today. As you progress through the book, I will give you support to overcome binge eating or problem overeating for the long term.

Mindfulness can help you to:

- Eat all foods in moderation.

- Enjoy food.

- Be at peace with food, ourselves and the world.

- Notice, and deal with emotions that are troublesome or triggering.

- Improve your self-image.

- Establish alternative methods to self-soothe, and comfort yourself that don't involve massive amounts of food.

- Develop healthier habits to deal with stress, anxiety or negative emotions.

- Become more resilient.

- Improve your quality of sleep.

- Enjoy food without feeling guilty or out of control.

- Appreciate your body.

- Deal with cravings.

- Enjoy movement.

- Accept thoughts and feelings without harsh judgements.

- Devise an individualised eating plan right for you.

- Move away from 'all or nothing 'thinking.

- Accept your body and appearance.

- Improve your relationships with others.

Mindfulness is not a quick fix solution. But it works. Consider this phrase: 'consistency trumps intensity'. (1) This means that sticking to a gentle but effective program will work. Many of us have got excited about a strict diet that made many wild promises – the more restrictive the diet, the more hopeful we were. Or, we got all pumped about a rigorous exercise regime that ended up making us feel worn out and depleted. Both super-charged, high-intensity approaches are not sustainable in the longer term. By the very nature of this unsustainability, we would inevitably 'fail' at the diet or not have the energy to keep up with the exercise regimen.

A consistent program will work because we can sustain it. It is more realistic to commit to a mindful walk for twenty minutes each day, mindful eating and some meditative activities because we can sustain these approaches. If we miss one activity one day, it's no big deal, just do it the next day. There are fewer highs and lows. Later, we will look at why binge eaters are attracted to these intense, novel diets or exercise programs but for now please accept that 'consistency trumps intensity'.

Finally, mindfulness is not a substitute for medical advice but can be a tool to support you with binge eating, compulsive over-eating, food addiction or emotional eating. If you use this book, I would encourage you to share the practices you have found helpful with your therapist to ensure they are compatible with your treatment.

This is Not a Diet Book

We cannot fix weight with diets. That statement may puzzle you but bear with me. You may lose weight by following a strict diet for a period, but what happens when you reach or get close to your target weight and you come off the diet? For most people, the weight creeps back. Often, the dieter will end up heavier than they were before the diet. We can only sustain diets in the short term. Diets provide a superficial fix to a problem that is much deeper than restricting food. This book uses mindfulness techniques and practical strategies to get to the heart of your battle with food.

This book is not a diet book. I do not advocate any diet plan, other than a balanced and nutritious eating plan that comprises all the major food groups. I encourage you to enjoy your food and eat the food you like. Stop dieting or starving yourself; under-eating can cause the 'dam to bust' when you eat and can lead to a binge.

Feast–Famine

These two words sum up the trap that we can get caught in:

- Feast–we over-eat or use food as our only comfort in life.

- Famine–we panic about weight piling on and find a restrictive diet to follow.

- Feast – we feel miserable and deprived so we overeat.

  Freedom–I hope to guide you in finding freedom, peace and balance around eating.

I would suggest that you avoid any eating plans or styles of eating that advocate cutting out entire food groups. Avoid any extreme eating plans. Diets that comprise fasting, clean eating, cleansing, detoxing or comprise only juices or raw food. These types of eating plans usually make extravagant promises and are restrictive diets under the disguise of so-called healthy eating.

Do not skip meals and eat when you are hungry. Avoid getting overly hungry. I will encourage you to tune in with your body to identify hunger and satiety. If you have forgotten what hunger or fullness feels like, I will give you guidance on how to re-discover these sensations.

Let go of rules and restrictions.

This might be a frightening prospect. In the early days and weeks, you might need to follow some guidelines, but these are not rules. Ultimately you will want to trust your natural desire to eat – when to eat, what to eat and how much to eat. This will take time. I will use the analogy of learning how to ride a bicycle to illustrate this point. When you first get on a bicycle, you wobble and lose balance; you need stabilisers and a supportive adult to help you stay upright and moving. In the early days of learning how to eat in a way that is nourishing and feels safe, you will need some support. The suggestions I make on managing cravings, dealing with trigger foods or avoiding binges, are just suggestions intended to guide and support. Use them in the early days as you begin to discover how it feels to be genuinely hungry, comfortably full and you are establishing healthy eating habits. You might wobble and lose balance sometimes, but by being mindful and paying attention, you will readjust and find the balance you need. Be patient, it takes time, practice and some slips along the way.

By following a plan of eating nutritious food regularly, your body will get back into balance and it will be easier to sense genuine hunger and fullness. These sensations may have become skewed because of very restrictive eating patterns.

If your doctor has advised you to lose weight due to a serious health issue, your weight will stabilise at a natural set point, as you practise the behaviours outlined in this book. Also, bear in mind that there are lots of skinny unhealthy people around. Focus on health and well-being. Try not to obsess about a number on the bathroom scale; focus on your behaviours around food and movement and over time, the weight will stabilise. Let go of striving and beating yourself up. Be patient.

If you are new to meditation or feel it is not for you, I will give you support. I offer guided meditations, as some people may find it difficult to just sit and observe their thoughts. It can be discouraging to feel that you are continuously struggling with thoughts. I will not ask you to empty your mind of thoughts. Everyone no matter how experienced at meditating will have thoughts come and go. That's how our minds work. The guided meditations will make it a little easier to accept that thought come and go.

You cannot do mindfulness 'wrong'. Just get into the flow of the short, simple practices regularly.

How to Use This Book

I structure this book as an eight-week program. I used this structure in my previous book *Mindfulness for Stress and Anxiety*. Many of my readers commented on how this structured approach supported them in their practice. Therefore, I hope that this eight-week program will be just as beneficial in this context.

I divide the book into eight chapters, one chapter for each week, each with seven sections. I would suggest that you start at the chapter for week one and spread the book out over eight weeks, reading one short section each day and completing one chapter per week. You can then use the book as a resource to turn back to when you feel you need a refresher on certain aspects.

An audio meditation will accompany each chapter to give you extra support. The meditations are on themes related to the particular chapter they accompany. I also include guided meditations to help you if you feel you have a binge coming on and to provide some comfort in dealing with feelings after a binge. I aim to give you maximum support in overcoming the difficulties you may be experiencing.

I design the book to offer you daily inspiration, guidance, helpful tips, structure, and support as you read it over the next eight weeks. By spreading the readings and exercises out over this period, you are giving yourself the optimum chance of incorporating these practices into your life. The practices will help to reveal and adjust deep-rooted thinking and behaviour around food.

This book will have fresh ideas to support you with making the changes you want to make to your eating behaviours right the way to the end of the book, so keep reading. I have spread the techniques out throughout the chapters and each chapter will have different tips and hints to incorporate mindfulness practices and supporting behaviours into your life.

Remember, mindfulness is a practice; that means that we need to practise it, not just read about it. I aim to make this practice accessible and practical. I want to give you maximum support to find peace with food, your emotions and body.

Each day I will prompt you to do these three activities:

- Read the relevant section from this book for the day you are on. If you miss a day, just catch up where you left off.

- Listen to the guided meditation for that week, once a day.

- Note down your observations in a journal. I will give you prompts to think about. The record you keep in your journal will help you see patterns of thoughts, feelings and behaviours.

There will be suggestions for additional activities to support you. You can pick and choose what resonates with you, but I would ask that you commit to the above three activities as a minimum to get started.

The beauty of a mindfulness practice is that much of it relates to how we do our usual activities rather than doing lots of extra things. I will urge you to reflect on certain attitudes or ways of being, which will impact on how you relate to food, your body, yourself and others.

Above all, commit to treating yourself with care, kindness and acceptance.

The Importance of Care, Compassion, and Kindness

Many binge eaters talk of a feeling of emptiness. Consuming massive amounts of foods is the only comfort for this lonely, sad part of themselves. The foods used are usually foods such as chocolate, biscuits, (cookies) sweets, baked goods, crisps (chips), ice-cream, or takeaway food. It's an empty promise, though. When there is physically no room to cram in more food, the emotional ache still goes on, with the false hope of fulfilment next time. We will, therefore, spend some time working through troubling emotions.

By beginning to practise some self-care, compassion and kindness you can give yourself what you can't find at the bottom of a crisp bag. Compassion, care, and kindness need to be practised. They don't just happen. You need to make some minor changes and build some new habits to nurture and soothe yourself without food. This means caring for your mind, your body, and your emotional self.

Fear around food or anxiety about being tempted to binge sets off the fight-or-flight response. This is an ancient chain reaction that takes place in our body to prepare us to deal with a threat. The body releases hormones such as cortisol. These stress hormones give us the energy to run or fight back. Unfortunately, cortisol has been shown to increase appetite and decrease feelings of satiety. We need to calm this stress response. By being compassionate with yourself, you will help yourself physiologically to off-set the anxiety that you might experience around food.

If we use the analogy of taming a wild animal; the animal will only be more savage if we beat it. Eventually, it might become submissive but be resentful and distrusting. If we are consistent, gentle and patient we will tame the animal. We will earn its respect and trust. By treating your problem eating with consistency, patience and compassion, you will tame those raging cravings and urges and trust and respect yourself.

There will be lots of practical ideas in this book on how to build in practices that provide the sustenance and nourishment you need.

The Inner Critic

The inner critic is that voice that is usually going on in the background. It might use phrases that a parent used or a harsh teacher from your school days. It might sound like a judgemental ex-partner or critical sibling. The phrases might be those such as, who do you think you are?', 'you aren't qualified to do that', and 'you're too old / too fat / too young / too inexperienced / too big / too small. The inner critic might take you down the supermarket aisle where all the sweets, biscuits and cakes are saying something like: 'go for it, what's the point anyway, you'll always be fat'.

If you are or have been someone who lives in a larger body you will have experienced the bias that society has against larger people. Sadly, research shows that family and friends will show the most bias against the larger people in their lives. You may have experienced relatives or friends judgements about your weight or size. You may have received praise for losing weight and either an embarrassed silence or admonishment for being heavier. I have known people who have avoided friends and family because of shame about weight gain. These experiences feed our harsh inner critic.

The inner critic is like a radio on in the background. You might tune into various radio stations. There might be a radio station that is telling you are fat and ugly or another one pointing out all your flaws. You can tune in or tune out. By being aware of the inner critic, we can make this conscious choice.

At present, the inner critic might operate at such a low background level that you are hardly aware of it, but the inner critic is running the show. Let's use the analogy of a bus; passengers and driver. Imagine these thoughts, which are just conditioned programming from the past, are the passengers and you are the driver. As the driver, your route is being dictated by these unruly, critical passengers, you are not sure where you are headed next. When you face the passengers and see that they are just passengers, they do not dictate the route; you can get on with the driving. Taking your bus in the direction you want to go.

We will talk more about the inner critic and how you can deal with it, as the book progresses.

Journaling

I have asked you to commit to keeping a journal over the next eight weeks as you work through this book. You can use your journal in the following ways:

- Spot patterns and habits around your eating behaviours.

- Identify the feelings and emotions that come up.

- Note how you relate to your body.

- Record how you use your time.

- Make observations on the quality of your relationships.

- Identify what inspires and motivates you.

- Pour out your feelings onto paper–especially challenging feelings.

- Make a note of particular memories or connections that come up from your past that impact on your eating behaviour.

- Make a note of intentions and commitments to your well-being.

The act of handwriting stimulates a part of the brain called the Reticular Activating System (RAS). This system filters everything you are aware of and gives greater importance to the thing you are focusing on at that moment. The act of writing will help in personal awareness and insights into your behaviour, motivations and intentions. Just to clarify: by 'writing' I mean the old-fashioned way, with a pen and paper.

A Note to Male Readers

Later in the book, I discuss the pressure women are under to look a certain way. Men also, increasingly, have more pressure on them to attain an idealised appearance; to have ripped muscles and a six-pack. Men's so-called 'fitness' is a big industry. Many weird and not so wonderful shakes, powders and extreme exercise regimes can skew men's' relationship with food and with their bodies.

Sometimes the severity of binge eating can be dismissed by remarks such as, 'He loves his food.' Or 'He's a big boy!' with a note of admiration and amusement. This attitude masks the misery of binge eating and the pain behind it. Sometimes it is only when the physical side effects of overeating get to be unbearably severe that a man will seek help. I know of a case in which a man in his thirties was overeating so much that he developed an extreme form of reflux, which meant he was waking up surrounded in vomit each morning. Knowing this was not right, he sought help from his doctor. It is sad that the problem has to get so extreme before someone seeks treatment.

For men too, food can become the only way they deal with powerful emotions. In week 4, I discuss how men are not given enough outlets in our society to express emotion and process it. The message boys get growing up is to be strong and show no weakness. This is as damaging as the messages little girls get, to be good and not get angry.

The figures show that more women seek help for eating issues than men. This does not mean that there are fewer men with problem eating, just that fewer seek help.

I hope this book is useful to you and also I would encourage you to ensure you get the support you need, talk to a trusted friend or family member or have a chat with your health professional.

Thank you for your trust and I wish you well.

Summary

This introduction will give you a flavour of the book. If it appeals to you, I look forward to guiding you in getting started next week.

To prepare for week one:

Get a notebook to use as a journal. Any notebook will do. It need not be perfect. This is just for your use and does not need to a beautifully presented journal.

Commit to these three activities each day.

1. Read the daily section.

2. Complete an entry in your journal.

3. Listen to a meditation each day.

There will be additional suggested activities to try out. Use those that appeal to you, but try to complete the three core actions each day.

Also in week 1, I will ask you to complete a quick exercise that requires the colours green, orange and red–any pens, pencils or crayons will do.

Consider your hopes, dreams and motivation in embarking on this journey. We will delve deeper into this next week.

A heartfelt thank you for staying with me this far, I admire your courage and determination.

I wish you health, happiness, and peace.

Week One

Getting Started

Food reveals our connection with the earth. Each bite contains the life of the sun and the earth...we can see and taste the whole of the universe in a piece of bread. **Thich Nhat Hanh.**

Maria

Maria busied herself about the kitchen. She loved days like this. It was a Saturday afternoon; the sun illuminated the south-facing kitchen. She could hear her young sons, Joe and Ben, laughing in the living room as they played Minecraft together. Sam, Maria's husband, was out in the garden setting up tables and hanging up birthday bunting for Joe's seventh birthday. Maria decided she would be 'good' today; no cake, no ice cream, no sweets, no biscuits.

Maria sipped on iced water as she laid out the pastel-coloured cupcakes in their pretty, spotted cases. Everyone would start arriving at 2 pm, Maria anticipated the excitement of the party, and she had put so much effort into planning games and making up party bags. She kept telling herself she would be fine. She promised herself she would not even have one nibble of the party treats she was laying out on trays ready for her young guests.

She felt her stomach rumble, but she ignored it, determined to stick to her diet. She had blown it last Saturday. Today

---

would be different. Today she was determined to get through the day without letting herself down again.

1. Commitment

This week I would like you to consider why you want to do something about your problem overeating. Why do you want to stop these behaviours?

The reason I ask you to do this is to get clarity about your motivations to begin this mindfulness journey. If you are clear about the 'why' there will be more chance you will commit to the practice, especially in the early days and weeks.

Our western minds like to have clear intentions, so this exercise in getting clear about what is motivating you, is an acknowledgement of this need. Gradually, you will feel the benefits of mindfulness and this initial 'why' will become less important. For now, being clear about your own personal 'why' will help you get started.

This is your personal journey. There are no 'shoulds' in this book. You chose what resonates with you. Being clear about what is motivating you, helps to further personalise this process of making mindfulness practices an integral part of your life. The following are just some ideas to consider:

Breaking Free From Diets.

You may feel you want freedom from the negative mental and physical effects of diets focussed on weight loss. Typically dieting follows this pattern: a vicious cycle of starting a diet, restricting food, feeling deprived, craving food, giving in to the craving, feeling guilty about indulging, then starting the diet all over again. You may want to break free from this trap.

To help get you started, we will look at some health and well-being issues that the diet culture has caused. Later we will look at the issues around overeating.

Restrictive diets cause:

- Feelings of frustration and failure.
- Confusion about what is actually healthy.
- Loss of trust in our ability to choose the amount and type of food that is best for us as individuals.
- Lowered self-esteem.
- An inability to recognise the bodily sensations of hunger and satiety.
- An obsession with numbers, portions, weight and size, that takes our attention away from enjoyable activities or meaningful work or projects.
- Imbalances in hormones and blood sugar levels.
- Feelings of weakness and fatigue.
- Feelings of lack of self-control or willpower.
- Production of stress hormones which promote weight gain and are linked to type-2 diabetes and cancer.
- Increased risk of problems related to inadequate nutrition, including increased sensitivity to fibre rich foods, decreased bone mineral density or deficiencies in vitamins and minerals.
- Increased risk of developing eating disorders.

- Impaired concentration and cognitive function.

The Minnesota Starvation Experiment carried out in November 1944 showed the effects of a semi-starvation diet. (1). Thirty-six male volunteers were put on a diet of 1.570 calories per day, for six months (for some readers this might seem like quite a generous calorific allowance). The men showed a decrease in stamina, body temperature and heart rate. They obsessed about food, reporting that they dreamed about it and fantasised about eating. The men reported feelings of fatigue, irritability, depression, apathy and a reduction in mental ability. Many of these men developed eating disorders.

Ultimately restrictive, fad diets don't work. More recently, Traci Mann shows why diets don't work in her book, *Secrets from the Eating Lab*. (2). Interestingly, her findings echo those of The Minnesota Starvation Experiment, for example, dieters become obsessed with food.

On the flip side, let's look at the problems overeating might cause:

Shame

Due to the messages, we may have internalised about our bodies and diets we may feel deep shame and distress about overeating. Shame is a deeply disturbing emotion and we will discuss it more later in the book.

Fear

We may fear food, or fear certain foods. This can be experienced as stress and anxiety which ignites the stress response. The stress hormones that are released can increase the appetite and decrease feelings of fullness. Mindfulness can help interrupt this stress response and help us feel calmer around food.

Overeating can disrupt the appetite.

Mindfulness helps us to be more aware of when, what and how overeating plays itself out in your life. By being more mindful of your bodily sensations you will cue into natural signs of hunger and fullness.

Nausea and digestive discomfort; overeating makes us feel sick and uncomfortable.

You may suffer from indigestion or conditions such as Irritable Bowel Syndrome. You might struggle with gas or bloating. Eating slowly and mindfully will help ease these problems. After a binge, you may have excessive sweating, a racing pulse, sore gums and a swollen tongue.

Problem eating comes with an array of social and mental issues, including a higher risk of depression and anxiety and problems such as avoiding social events and intimacy. This can lead to feelings of isolation and loneliness.

Overeating causes feelings of sluggishness and affects energy levels.

Reactive hypoglycaemia means that the blood sugar level drops shortly after eating if you are constantly overeating, this sluggish, below par feeling will be a constant companion.

Overeating is associated with the following health issues: Type 2 diabetes, heart problems, high blood pressure, high cholesterol, joint and back problems and fertility issues. There is some debate about this correlation. Which comes first, the health issue or the eating issue? For example, pre-diabetics or undiagnosed diabetics will have huge swings in blood sugar levels. This can lead people to binge eat to ease the symptoms of dramatic drops in blood sugar. They will then gain weight. If you haven't had a check-up recently, I would urge you to have a medical, to see if there are biological reasons for your urge to overeat.

What we need then is a balanced approach to weight, food and exercise. We see that fad diets or semi-starvation do not work and we see that chronic overeating or binge eating is detrimental to our physical, mental and emotional health. Finding peace with food, our bodies and our emotions, can work to achieve that balance.

A note about body fat.

If your doctors are concerned about the amount of weight you are carrying, this might be your motivation to eat more mindfully. Please check with your doctor. Many binge eaters judge themselves harshly and have a history of restrictive dieting that has contributed to a skewed relationship with food. If you have been told to lose weight due to a serious health issue, by changing your behaviour and living more mindfully, your weight will level out. To reiterate, this book is not a diet book. We will focus on basic, common-sense health principles. I would urge you to consult with a nutritionist to get an eating plan suitable for your particular needs.

Your motivations to overcome binge eating might be to:

- Sleep through the night without being bothered by indigestion or food cravings.
- Enjoy more sports or physical activity.
- Feel more energetic and enjoy life.
- Have peace of mind.
- Enjoy social occasions without worrying about food.
- Feel more comfortable physically and emotionally.
- Feel more connected with others.
- Feel whole, loved and complete just as you are – not because you are thinner or smaller.
- Gain control over finances – eating enormous amounts of food can be expensive.

These are not fixed goals or concrete expectations; they are an indicator of how you are thinking now. Later in the book, we will talk about letting go and non-striving. For now, you can sit easy with these motivations. Let's let go of expectations and see how it all unfolds.

No matter what size you are or what is motivating you, I would urge you to accept yourself as you are. You don't have to wait to get 'fixed' to enjoy life. Let go of forcing yourself to restrict food, exercise frantically, or shame yourself into getting thin. You are an amazing, unique, and beautiful human being just as you are.

As we come to the end of this section, take a moment to reflect on what has resonated with you. Take a breath in, close your eyes and put your right hand over your heart. Tune in to what is going through your mind and what emotions you are feeling. Spend a few moments reflecting on your hopes and wishes as you begin this course in mindfulness. If any self-judgement comes up, let it go.

Summary for day one:

Today you have reflected on your motivation to begin a mindfulness practice. This is just for you. Remember, I am not asking you to set goals or have concrete outcomes.

This record will help keep you motivated and will be an interesting reflection to look back on later in your mindfulness journey. Your motivations might change as you go forwards.

Pour out your feelings about your struggles, hopes, dreams and fears.

Well done, on taking the first step. Confronting your binge eating takes courage and commitment. Take a moment to appreciate these qualities in yourself.

2. Compulsive Overeating, Binge Eating, Binge Eating Disorder and Emotional Eating.

We all overeat sometimes. Most people have eaten to excess at Christmas or during other holiday celebrations when the principal focus of the celebration is food. However, compulsive overeating, binge eating, Binge Eating Disorder and emotional eating have distinctive characteristics that profoundly affect sufferers' well-being and health.

Emotional Eating

Eating and emotions are closely interwoven. We all eat for comfort from time to time and there is nothing wrong with that. However, emotional eaters use food as their dominant method to deal with emotions. Emotional eaters attempt to escape emotions by shutting down emotions completely or feeling overwhelming emotions. Just as we can't fix our weight with diets, we can't fix emotional hunger with food. Food satisfies physical hunger, but not emotional hunger.

By being mindful of emotions and accepting them, you can move forward. By identifying patterns of behaviour and emotional responses, we can deal with cravings at a deeper level. There will be much more on dealing with emotions in Week 4.

This book will be of help to anyone who is an emotional eater. Most of us associate emotion and food. I associate the smell and taste of potato cakes with childhood memories of being in my grandmother's kitchen where I felt warm and safe. An enjoyable meal is pleasurable. Food is associated with joyous occasions such as birthdays, winter celebrations and anniversaries. However, an emotional eater is someone who takes these natural connections to extremes.

Reasons for emotional eating:

- The need for comfort.
- To escape painful feelings.
- Trauma.
- Lack of support.
- Difficulties in coping with life.

This book can help with learning how to deal with emotions healthily. The book, *The Emotional Mind* by Lewis David also available from WinsPress.com will give you further help in dealing with troubling emotions.

There will be much more on emotional eating later in this book.

Binge Eating and Compulsive Overeating.

Perhaps your binges are infrequent and relatively harmless; however, if you are bothered by your own behaviour around food, you can gain some control that is not based on willpower. Perhaps you feel that once you eat, it is extremely difficult to stop. Later, we will look at the causes of problems with eating. As you work through this book, you will learn about exercises and practices to incorporate into daily life to help break these urges to binge or overeat.

If you feel that you are a compulsive eater and that you have fallen into poor habits around food, this book can help you. By approaching eating and food more mindfully and adopting the suggestions and tips in this book, you will gently reconfigure your habits to eat more healthfully. If you are overeating mindlessly, this book will help get you back on track.

Binge Eating Disorder

BED is characterised by a sense of loss of control over food, particularly highly palatable foods such as sugary, fatty or very salty foods. Over the years, the sense of loss of control may fade and the binge eater plans the binges; giving an illusion of control. People with BED will eat when they are not hungry and will experience deep shame, guilt and regret after a binge eating episode. Often, the binge will be in secret. There is nothing sociable or celebratory about this pattern of eating.

Feelings of an altered state of consciousness may accompany the binge–almost like a trancelike state. Often there is a distraction during the binge such as television or loud music; this acts to distance the person from what they are doing.

In 2013, the American Psychiatric Association recognised BED and listed the following diagnostic criteria:

- There are frequent objective binges – at least once a week.
- Extreme methods of weight control including excessive use of laxatives, intensive exercise or extreme dieting or fasting.

- A deep concern with weight and shape.
- Not be significantly underweight.

Dr Christopher Fairburn, an authority on eating disorders, describes these diagnostic criteria as 'arbitrary'. (1). He points out that what really matters is that binge eating is interfering with a person's physical health or quality of life.

If you are suffering from BED, I would urge you to speak with a health professional and get support.

You can use this book to complement your treatment. Talk to your health professional about taking this mindfulness-based approach to your binge eating. The insights you will get in your mindfulness practice will help clarify your triggers, responses and patterns of behaviour. I hope these insights will augment your treatment.

What Is A Binge?

Practitioners working with binge eaters categorise binges into:

1. Objective binges - Objective binges are episodes of extreme over-eating that run into thousands of calories in one sitting.

2. Subjective binges. - Subjective binges are when the food consumed is perceived to be a binge by the person eating it. For some people, eating two biscuits could be considered a binge.

What Causes Problem Eating?

You may wish to reflect on whether any of these possible causes apply to you:

Family background.

Often problem eating seems to run in families. This could be genetics or family habits and traditions. What were your parents' attitudes toward food? Was there any restriction or scarcity of food in your home when you were growing up? Do your siblings have any issues with food? In researching for this book I interviewed a woman in her fifties who reflected on her upbringing and how this affected her eating behaviours:

"Food was very tightly controlled in my home when I was a child. I was not allowed to help myself from the fridge or cupboards. My mother suffered from depression and would often stay in bed all day. My father worked as a travelling salesman and was usually away from home for days or weeks at a time. Weekends and holidays were the worst. I would wander about the house feeling hungry and sneak into the kitchen to 'steal' food. My mother would be furious if she caught me taking food.

When she got up late in the afternoon, she would make me tea and toast with biscuits. Then late in the evening, we would have a vast meal of processed food such as tinned meat and frozen chips. I would eat until I was bursting, as I had felt so hungry all day.

We never had fruit or fresh vegetables. We never had a proper breakfast or lunch. My mother had been a child during World War Two and told me stories of how her family had no food for days at a time. I remember how she would hoard food and she definitely had issues around eating. I feel that many of my problems stemmed from my family background.''

On the other hand, you may have grown up in a very permissive household where you got what you wanted with no restrictions or delay. There may have been no boundaries, and you never had to wait to get anything. This could build a pattern of impulsive behaviour and expectations of immediate gratification. Slowing down and being mindful of impulses and reactions can help highlight awareness of this issue.

Trauma.

Issues with food can develop after trauma for many reasons. Have you experienced any trauma in your life? Have you had support or treatment for this? Did your relationship with food or with your body change after a traumatic event?

Dieting.

We will talk more about this in the book. Have you followed diets or restrictive patterns of eating? When did you first start to diet? How do you feel when you are not on a diet? Have you been a member of diet clubs or programmes?

Depression.

Have you suffered from depression or frequent low mood? If you do feel depressed, I would urge you to talk to your medical professional. Do you eat more when you feel low? Do you feel trapped in a cycle of eating more when you feel low and then feeling depressed or down because of the amount you have eaten?

Substance Abuse.

Do you have any issues with heavy drinking or using drugs addictively? If so, get support from your doctor. Also, books such as *The 10 Day Alcohol Detox* and *Alcohol and You,* both by Lewis David and available from WinsPress.com, will be helpful.

Body Shaming.

Have you felt shame or deep dissatisfaction with your body and appearance? What sort of messages did you receive about your body as you were growing up? What sort of thoughts come into your mind when you look in the mirror? How do you feel about intimacy? Feeling shame about the body is not just a problem for women, increasingly more boys and men are struggling with these issues. I once worked with a middle-aged man I will refer to as, Gordon. This is what he shared with me:

"I always felt fat and unattractive. Everyone in my family was overweight as I was growing up. I was a shy teenager and didn't go out much. I went to university but found it hard to cope with the social pressure. I stayed at home to take care of my father. My mother had passed away in my

early twenties. I looked after my dad for ten years. My main comfort was food. I would take care of him during the day, clean and shop, and then in the evenings, I would just eat. The more I ate, the bigger I got, and I hated the way I looked. When my dad passed away it devastated me, I felt like I had nothing except food. I've never had a close personal relationship, as I have always felt too embarrassed about how I look. I feel very lonely and the only comfort I have is eating. It feels like I am trapped in a vicious cycle.''

Distinct Types of Binges.

The starvation binge – you have gone too long without food and you are ravenous. You binge because you have starved yourself all day.

The end of diet binge – you have endured hunger and restriction. You may or may not have got to your goal weight, but either way, you decide you are off the diet. You go for the food you have been denying yourself. The floodgates are open.

Feeling sad/low or sorry for yourself binge – this binge happens when we feel stressed, exhausted, upset or hormonal. We use food to comfort, reward or rebel.

Feeling body shame or disgust – we turn to food to comfort ourselves, to deal with uncomfortable emotions about our bodies.

The night-time binge – due to fatigue, boredom or to seek numbness.

The social binge – this could be a party, buffet, barbeque or lavish dinner. We eat more than we intended and feel uncomfortable.

The afternoon slump binge – we overeat food high in sugar, fat, salt and refined flour to fend off plummeting blood sugar levels or deal with exhaustion or boredom.

Emotional Eating.

In this book, we will look at four aspects of problem eating:

- Food
- Emotions.
- Self-esteem.
- Body image.

As we draw today's reading to a close, please go back and consider some questions posed in this section. Make a few notes in your journal about the patterns of your binges or episodes of overeating. Reflect on some reasons you feel you started to overeat or have binged. Remember to do this with an attitude of gentleness on yourself.

3. Avoiding Binges.

Later, we will look at the reality of food addiction. We will also learn about the power of ingrained habits that trigger food binges.

EAT! Eat well and often. Don't starve yourself, it will backfire. Food cravings could be the result of a lack of nutrition. Cravings are indicators that we can notice and honour. We are not pushing cravings away. Like troubling emotions, cravings are signals that we can be aware of and take some action on. Next week we will look in detail at a suggested plan of eating to ensure your body gets maximum nutrition.

In the early days and weeks of recovery from problem overeating, it can be tricky to work out which cravings are okay and which cravings might lead to a binge. By being consciously aware and keeping a record in your journal, you will spot which foods you can eat and enjoy and which foods lead to a binge. No food is banned. By being more switched on about your own personal reactions to foods you can work out ways of having your cake and eating it. For example, only keep individual portion sizes at home or have cake when you go out for coffee. There will be more on this later.

You might feel compelled to eat to deal with your emotions. We will discuss emotional eating more in Week 5. This mix of the availability of trigger foods we know we will binge on plus feeling emotionally vulnerable, nutritionally deficient and or physically tired, stressed or drained is a combination that will probably lead to a binge.

By being mindful of the following, we can avoid falling into the trap of binge eating:

- Trigger foods.
- Food quality.
- Emotions.

- Context (coming home from work/ unstructured time).

By engaging in mindfulness practices, you can have more insight into your motivations, feelings, and responses. By regularly considering how you feel emotionally or by practising a body scan, (I will explain the body scan in Day 5.) you can be more in touch with your feelings and needs.

For example, in your work life, you might usually plough on through the afternoon, dismissing or ignoring your feelings. You might be vaguely aware of a sense of fatigue, but you override it with coffee and sugary snacks at work. You battle home in the traffic and arrive home exhausted and suffering from a big drop in blood sugar as a reaction to the sweets eaten at work. Your brain has been trained to take you to the fridge and find the most sugary, salty, or processed fat-filled snacks you can find. You are all set for a full-on binge.

By noticing about how you feel, acknowledging it, and dealing with it in healthful ways, you can avoid predictable triggers. By practising mindfulness the scenario above could look like this:

It's 3 pm at work. The office is busy and feels stuffy. You have noticed this as you stop and pause and look around you. You make a mental note of how you feel in your body and notice that you are holding your shoulders tight and they seem to have got higher. You do a neck roll and hear your neck creak. You open a window and take a few breaths of fresh air, stretch and move to the water machine and have a couple of glasses of water. You realise you are hungry and you keep some whole food snacks such as nuts, fruit, and wholegrain cereal bars in your drawer. You eat your snack mindfully, enjoying every morsel, and carry on working with renewed focus.

By taking a few minutes – even just seconds to be mindful and meet your needs appropriately and in a timely manner, you can avoid the hunger, exhaustion and pent up tension that seems to flood over you suddenly, at the end of a working day.

Some experts believe a food craving lasts between three to five minutes. We are all individuals and will experience food cravings differently. The craving *will* cease. Try to ride it out. In this way, you will be re-wiring the pleasure circuit in your brain. You will be re-educating your brain to feel the craving and let it pass without eating huge amounts of food.

- Be honest with yourself and clear out foods you know you will binge on. Alternatively, you could keep these foods in the house but only in moderate amounts. Avoiding trigger foods is not a pre-requisite to recovery, but it can make life easier, especially in the early days. If you have to leave the house to get binge foods, you might be less likely to binge. This will be different for each person.

On your mindfulness journey, you will identify these foods that cause you the most problem and you may decide not to keep them at home. We are not talking about abstinence forever; this strategy might only be needed as you begin to establish more balanced eating habits.

If you know you will lose control around a cream trifle and end up eating the entire thing yourself, get it out of the house. You are not at war with food; you are making decisions and choices that help you end the struggle with food and eating. Making it more difficult to get foods you know are triggers for you can help you feel more comfortable and safer in your kitchen.

If you can have a small amount of your favourite food without losing control, try only keeping pre-portioned amounts of the foods such as a single slice of cake or mini-chocolate bars. If eating these sets you off on a chocolate eating rampage, then it might be best to avoid having these foods for now.

For some people, it might be best to avoid keeping large amounts of cakes or chocolates at home. However, they have sweets when they go out for a coffee or a meal. In this way, they can enjoy these foods and don't feel deprived. It's a very personal choice.

The key thing is to do what gives you the most peace with food. If you feel agitated and can't rest until you eat the entire box of chocolates, then it will probably be more comfortable for you to avoid routinely keeping large boxes of chocolate at home. Keep it as an occasional food to eat in moderation.

By being mindful of shopping and eating habits, you can be aware of the foods you crave. If you binge, make a note in your journal of the circumstances, type of food, time of day, your emotions and physical sensations. Don't beat yourself up about the binge; look on it as an opportunity to gain more information about your eating habits. Write yourself a letter expressing kindness and forgiveness to yourself, to read after a binge. If this is difficult, pretend you are writing it for a dear friend.

Emotions and binging.

Later in the book, I will talk more detail about the role emotions can play in problem overeating.

For now, I would like you to reflect on the emotions that can cause you to binge. This will be different for everyone. You might binge when you are depressed or you might compulsively overeat when life is going well and you are intensely happy.

In your journal draw a green circle, an orange circle, and a red circle.

In the green circle write all the emotions you have when you feel okay around most foods – this could be emotions such as feeling loved, contented or peaceful.

In the orange circle write all the emotions you feel when you are feeling like a binge might be coming on – this could be frustrated, stressed or worried. Perhaps, the emotions for you might be less intense, such as feeling flat, bored or a bit low.

In the red circle write the emotions that in your experience you know will definitely lead to a full-scale binge – this could be feeling furious, rejected or fearful. This will be different for everyone. Some people might binge on 'high' emotions. They might binge when they feel elated, super-excited and over-joyed.

If you are not sure, take time over the next few days and weeks to be curious about the link between your emotions and binging. When you feel you have more information, return to this exercise and complete it.

If you can complete it now, be mindful of what is in each circle. If you feel you are experiencing emotions in the orange or red circles, take some mindful action. You might want to turn to the tips coming up on how to deal with cravings or the urge to binge.

As you progress through the book, there will be further help in dealing mindfully with emotions that could lead you to a binge.

How To Deal With An Urge To Binge - Some 'First-Aid' Strategies.

- As you stand looking in the fridge and you can see the food, you know you will lose control with; the first thing to do is **walk away from the fridge.** If you are not genuinely hungry and food tempts you, know it will lead to a binge; get out of the kitchen, and away from the fridge. You can then use some following techniques to focus your attention on something other than food until the craving passes.

- When you have walked away from the food, sit down comfortably and take a few breaths. Put your right hand on your heart and breathe into your heart. Breathe in compassion for yourself. Keep a spirit of curiosity about your feelings in the moment. Ask yourself some simple questions such as are you thirsty, are you genuinely hungry, do you need someone to talk to; are you feeling some powerful emotion? What do you need right now? Listen to the answers and take some action if needed – fetch some water, eat a nourishing snack if you are hungry, ring a friend or pour out your emotion in your journal.

- Using your dominant hand touch the tip of your forefinger and the tip of your thumb together. Imagine the finger as the past and the thumb as the future, the pressure between is the present. Focus on the present.

- Take a moment to close your eyes and imagine leaves floating down a stream. Each leaf is a craving, just floating away.

- Listen to the guided meditation I have prepared to help in this acute situation of being tempted to binge. This can be found at the beginning of Week 2.

- As a quick remedy, I have recommended the use of the essential oil of peppermint. This has worked well for people I have advised. Use top-grade natural essential oil. Put a drop on your palms, rub them together, and breathe in the fresh peppermint aroma. This will lift feelings of fatigue, encourage clarity of thinking, and interrupt the desire to eat when you are not hungry. (Not recommended if you are pregnant. Be careful not to get any oil in your eyes or around the nose – it will sting,)

- Think of some appealing activities to turn to instead of binging. List things you adore doing and you see as a treat. Make it easy for yourself to turn to these quickly, with minimal preparation. For example, keep an engrossing mystery novel somewhere easy to pick up or keep some heavenly bath oils within easy reach to treat yourself to an aromatic bath – whatever you feel will work for you. Make it easy for yourself to find something quick, accessible and enjoyable to do instead of binging. If you are exhausted, it can just seem like too much effort to get involved in an engrossing activity that could take your mind off food. Have a nap if you need to. Keep a bank of ideas ready to absorb your attention.

- Write yourself a letter reminding yourself of all the reasons you don't want to binge. Keep this letter to re-read during an episode of being tempted to binge.

- A quick remedy you could try is the power pose. The power pose or wonder woman pose comes from the research carried out by Amy Cuddy.(1)

Ms Cuddy asserts that this pose can help lower cortisol and increase testosterone. Balancing the hormones in this way can help you feel more in control of your behaviour and more peaceful:

Stand with your feet well planted on the floor and apart with your hands on your hips, your arms bend outwards. Breathe deeply through your nose for two minutes. Then see how you feel. Be mindful of your feelings before and after practising the pose. If it has helped, focus on this to instil this behaviour as a response when confronted with a craving. If you feel silly doing this, engage your inner child, and have a giggle at yourself. It's okay to see the funny side. This can take the misery out of the cravings or the urge to binge.

- Identify your emotions and work out ways to get what you need without using food as the first go-to activity to help you feel more comfortable. Refer to your completed traffic lights exercise to remind yourself of the emotions that could trigger you to binge. We will go into much more depth on emotions in Week 4. For now, if you do feel upset or down you could consider options such talking with a friend, getting a hug, getting out into nature, breathing deeply for a few moments, doing the guided meditation for this week, writing in your journal, gentle movement or stretching, a few minutes on a favourite screen-based activity (avoid triggering images relating to diets or thinness), writing wish lists such as places you would like to visit or write a gratitude list.

- Delay, don't deny – by this, I mean to say something to yourself along the lines of: "I won't eat this (name food) now but I can have it some other time…'' or "Okay but not today." If you know in your heart-of-hearts that you will eat the whole box of brownies, for example, promise yourself one brownie next time you go out for coffee, in a safer environment.

- If you are faced with a craving, you cannot physically remove yourself from practice observing the thought. You can't force the thoughts away but be a witness to the thoughts. Remind yourself that you are not the thought, you can just watch it come and go. I know this is hard. That's why I have listed lots of practical strategies above to get you started.

Over time, you will develop new responses to cravings. You realise that just because you have a craving, you do not have to give in to it unless you want to. Dr Judson Brewer describes the 'cycle of desire in his book: *The craving Mind.(*2) He describes how we can change how we relate mentally to these objects of desire by practising looking at the thought but not giving in to the craving. By being overwhelmed by the craving and giving in to it, we perpetuate this reward cycle and it continues to be difficult to deal with cravings. By detaching ourselves from the craving and becoming a dispassionate observer, we can change this undesired behaviour.

- Take some time this week to write yourself a letter to read when you are tempted to binge. Keep the letter somewhere handy. In the letter write all the things you admire about yourself, list all the reasons you want to get well and stop binging, list the non-food treats you have ready to turn to and give yourself permission to eat if you are hungry. Read the letter when you feel you want to binge.

If this seems like a lengthy list, the following acronym might help to remind you of the key points in dealing with a craving: R.I.D.E.

- **R**emove yourself from the temptation, if possible.
- **I**nvolve yourself in an engaging activity.
- **D**ecide if you really are hungry and eat if you need to.
- **E**valuate how you are feeling and what you really need in this moment. This might be a snack, or connection with friends, or a nap, water, or some gentle movement.

If you do binge, let's focus on harm reduction:

- Slow down, eat less frantically.
- Breathe slowly between each bite.
- Pay attention to the taste and texture of the food.
- Pay attention to the thoughts and feelings you have as you eat.
- Eat nourishing foods, such as nuts or dried fruits. These will satisfy you more quickly and although they are rich foods, they are full of nutrients.

- Talk yourself through what you are doing. This will raise awareness and slow you down. For example: *"I am putting the chocolate in my mouth. It is melting and has turned to liquid in my mouth. I am swallowing the chocolate and now I am reaching for another one..."*

Above all be compassionate with yourself. If the binge is shorter in duration or if you consume less food, that is progress.

Help! I've binged. What to Do After a Binge.

If you get overwhelmed and binge, please do not beat yourself up. Reflect on the circumstances of the binge and be mindful of what you could do differently in the future.

Be present with your feelings, even if they are distressing feelings such as regret or physical discomfort. Accept the feelings and know they will pass. The following are some practical tips to help deal with the aftermath of a binge:

- Sit for a few moments with your right hand over your heart, breathe in slowly and focus on love and acceptance of yourself.
- Listen to the guided meditation for after a binge.
- Read your letter to yourself for after a binge.
- Don't push yourself to over-exercise.
- Try some gentle movements or a walk to help relieve physical discomfort.
- Pour out your feelings onto paper. Use your journal to record how you feel.
- Talk to a trusted friend or family member.

- At the next regular mealtime have something to eat. Even if it is just a small snack. Don't skip a meal. This will just keep you on the binge/restrict merry-go-round.
- Do something pleasurable for your body such as a bubble bath.
- Have a nap. Binges can be emotionally draining.
- Listen to some soothing music.
- Wash your hair.
- Get busy with a project or chore around the house. Totally immerse yourself in what you are doing and don't rush.
- Get out into nature, a walk in a park, along a beach or in a forest can be soothing.

Today we have looked at what can be a key issue for many people, dealing with the temptation to binge. I hope you can pick out some practical steps you can take to manage this. Write what you think will be most helpful to you. This will assist you in committing those strategies to memory. By working through your craving to binge mindfully and with acceptance, you will take the power away from the binges. You learn that you can experience a craving without having to give in to a full-scale binge. This won't happen over-night – keep practising. If your binges become less intense, less frequent and shorter, you are progressing.

The effort it takes to ride out the urge to binge will be worth it. You will be re-wiring your brain to respond to these urges differently. You will be taking the power away from the craving bit by bit, each time you decide to treat yourself with respect and love by looking at the binge monster and staring it out.

4. Getting Started.

The following are some practical tips to support you as you go through the next eight weeks. There is a lot in this section, so please do not feel that you have to do everything today. Use this section as a resource. You can return to this section when you feel you need a reminder.

A key aspect of this programme is not to get over-hungry – eat when you need to.

Ask yourself - are you hungry?

Get in touch with how your body feels when you are hungry. Restrictive diets and binge eating have caused our eating to become disordered. Our cues to eat have become skewed. Mindfulness activities can help us reconnect with our body and emotions. When you feel that you want to eat, ask yourself if you are actually hungry? Does your stomach feel empty? How are your energy levels? Are you thirsty? Have a drink of water and then see how you feel. If you are hungry, go right ahead and eat. On Day 6 this week, we will look at mindful eating.

Eat regularly.

Do not skip meals or restrict your eating. Avoid going for lengthy periods without food. You will get over-hungry and this could trigger a binge. Avoid going for more than four hours during the day without food.

Plan.

Always have nutritious food that you enjoy in the fridge, freezer and cupboards. Have a well-balanced 'go-to' quick meal to fall back on if you get busy or fall behind in your schedule. Have a rough idea of what you will cook over the week and always shop with a shopping list. Shopping online is an excellent option, as it may be easier to avoid impulse buys of food on offer.

Stay hydrated.

Drink water. Avoid sweet carbonated drinks and too much caffeine.

Eat well during the day when you are expending the most energy.

Eat breakfast. By eating well during the day you avoid the trap of getting home at the end of the day, starving and the early evening 'snack' turns into a long evening of constant grazing on comfort foods. Get out of the habit of eating for comfort or relief from stress or difficult emotions in the evenings. I know this is easier said than done, but use the ideas in this book to cope with cravings, work through your emotions and practice self-care. If you wake up in the night, you might be tempted to binge. If you feel that hunger pangs will interrupt your sleep in the night, have a milky (plant-based or dairy depending on your preferences) drink before bed. This will help keep your blood sugar stable during the night. If you wake up have some warm herbal tea and read or do a boring task until you feel sleepy.

Eat food you enjoy.

Allow yourself to eat a range of foods as part of your daily eating plan. Complete denial of enjoyable foods could bring on a binge. Cutting out favourite foods encourages an 'all or nothing' attitude.

Plan enjoyable activities. - immerse yourself in a hobby, a DIY project or an engrossing book.

Avoid playing mental arithmetic with calories or points and don't store them up for later in the day.

Be aware of trigger situations.

Consider where you usually binge. Is it at home on your own? Do you lose control at parties or buffets? What sort of food do you feel you have no control over? How do you feel before a binge? Do you plan binges or do they seem to happen involuntarily?

Use your journal to record any observations or thoughts you have about the pattern of your binging. During this week, pay attention to your urges to binge. If you binge, be compassionate with yourself.

You can listen to my guided meditation to help you recover from a binge. See the binge experience as a source of information to help you better understand the binge habits you have developed over a long time. Accept that it will take time and attention to undo these habits.

Get rid of distractions when you are eating.

Avoid munching in front of a computer screen or a television set. Give your meal your complete attention.

Enjoy your food.

Don't ban *all* your favourite foods forever. As you practice mindful eating, investigate the foods you enjoy but. If you know you will lose control over a certain food, find a way to include it so that you won't feel deprived or pinpoint what you enjoy about a certain food and find a safer substitute. For example, if you know that once you eat crisps, you will eat an enormous family-sized bag in one sitting, avoid keeping the massive bags at home. What you might crave is the salty, crunchy texture – a few rice cakes with hummus could satisfy that or some air-popped popcorn with a shake of sea salt or nutritional yeast. You are making new habits to enjoy food in healthy ways. Alternatively, you could keep just an individual bag of crisps at home; eat them slowly with full enjoyment and attention.

Avoid eating out of the food container, for example, eating ice cream out of the box or biscuits (cookies) out of the packet. Portion out the food onto a plate or bowl.

Keep a food journal or app on your phone to track your eating. This might show up patterns of eating you have been unaware of. This is not to restrict eating, but to raise awareness. If an app causes you to feel like you are following a diet, get rid of the app.

Eat fibre rich foods that are nutritionally dense such as starchy vegetables and whole grains. Fill up on hearty soups and delicious salads topped off with beans or a sprinkle of nuts.

Be aware of possible trigger foods such as white bread, sweet and processed carbohydrates such as doughnuts and cakes. Enjoy nutritious and delicious fruits, dried fruit, nuts, wholegrain crackers, baked crispy vegetables or fruit-based desserts or crumbles to give yourself an indulgent pudding. White bread, sweets and processed carbohydrates can cause spikes in blood sugar levels, which could lead to a binge or episode of overeating.

In Week 2, we will look at food addiction. Manufacturers design these processed foods to keep us going back for more. Be aware of the foods that make you react in this way.

Remember, you are not on a diet. You are making choices beneficial to your mental well-being and health. You are seeking peace with food.

Eat at a table.

I once heard it said that the two pieces of furniture we should never get rid of are a table and a bookcase. If you haven't got a table, get one. If your table is covered in work-related items or general household debris, clear it off and set it up as an attractive dining area.

Eating at a table gives your brain the message you have eaten a meal. Avoid eating standing up, on the go or in the car. Make mealtimes as pleasant as possible. Set the table.

Put a flower or candle on the table. Use attractive crockery and utensils. Enjoy all aspects of the experience.

Cook or prepare your own food as much as possible. Keep takeaways and pre-prepared food as a treat. By preparing your own food, you know what has gone into it. This does not have to be elaborate. Simple one-pot dishes such as casseroles, curries, chillies and soups can be prepared in a slow cooker, ready to eat at the end of a busy day.

Depression and boredom

If you are eating because of depression or boredom, get some support with the depression. Find other ways to lift your mood, such as gentle movement, use of essential oils, music or nature. If you are bored, investigate ways to use your time productively and in an enjoyable way. Plan what you will do in unstructured time. Have you always nurtured a desire to paint, write, draw cartoons, or learn a language? Do you love reading historical romances or creating Pinterest boards?

Reduce stress

Stress drives up the levels of cortisol in the body. Cortisol can stimulate the appetite and lead to over-eating or a binge. Over the course of the next few weeks, notice the circumstances that cause your stress levels to rise. In Week 7 we will look at stress in more detail. Note down in your journal the aspects of your life, that you feel cause your stress or anxiety. You might need to make some changes or at least find different coping mechanisms to handle the stress. Mindfulness practices can help lower our perception of stress and manage anxiety in a more healthy way. There is more on this in my book *Mindfulness for Stress and Anxiety.*

Have a clear-out

Fridge and cupboards.

Avoiding trigger foods is not a pre-requisite of recovery from binge eating, but it makes the likelihood of not binging much higher, especially in the early days and weeks.

Look in your fridge and cupboards. Clear out any foods you know you will binge on. Having these foods readily available could sabotage your efforts in a moment of weakness. If you have lost touch with the foods that cause you the most problems, keep a food diary to help you see connections between your feelings, behaviour and food.

Enlist the support of your family. Tell them about your plans and ask them to remove foods you find problematic.

Be honest with yourself, clear out all your secret stashes in the bedroom, garage and top shelves. This will take courage. Be aware of any strong resistance or fear about this. Do what you can and be compassionate with yourself if you are not ready to do this. We will revisit these suggestions later in the book.

Clear out foods that are labelled low fat, diet or have reference to counting points. You are aiming to have an eating style that meets your nutritional needs, works for you and that is pleasurable but not addicting. Usually, these foods labelled low fat, diet or are part of a points system, are highly processed, are made from odd ingredients and contain pitifully small amounts. Also, consider how many times you have bought low-calorie biscuits or cakes but ate twice as many as you intended as you felt justified by the low-calorie label. This clear-out includes any mixes for diet shakes or teas that are marketed as aiding weight loss.

Your wardrobe.

Look in your wardrobe and pick out all the outfits and garments that you feel comfortable in and that you feel suit you. Give away any clothes you label as being your 'fat clothes' or 'thin clothes'. Only keep the clothes that fit you now. You could have a clothes swap with friends, sell clothes online or donate to a charity.

Enjoy the colour, texture and shape of your garments. An old-fashioned word to describe an attractive outfit is 'becoming'. Look on your clothing as helping you to 'become' who you really are. Dress for who you are, not to look like an image in a magazine or online.

Your bookshelf.

Look on your bookshelves or kindle. Give away or delete books that are diet orientated. Clear out any books on exercise that are focused on body image Keep your reading material focused on well-being and true health – including mental and emotional health.

Your bathroom.

Give the scales away, or at least put them out of sight. Drop the obsession with body weight. Your weight can fluctuate for many reasons including hormones, fluid intake, fluid retention or high salt intake. If you need to lose fat for medical reasons, your health professional will help you track your body fat using accurate devices. If you fear that your weight will creep up if you don't monitor it, weigh yourself once a week. You can do this at many pharmacies, so you don't really need to keep scales at home at all.

Go through your bathroom cabinet. Keep any medication recommended by your health professional and never stop any prescribed medications without medical advice. That being said, go through any pills or preparations you have bought that claim to help with weight-loss. Be mindful of your intentions around taking any non-prescribed medications. If you hope it will aid weight loss, question its benefit to you. If in doubt, discuss the medication with your local pharmacist or doctor.

Have a gratitude shower or bath

When you have a shower or bath, totally absorb yourself in the process. Bring to the experience a sense of gratitude for the hot water, the soap or shower gel. Most of all, cultivate a sense of gratitude for your body and all it does for you. Let go of ideas of what you think you should look like. Let go of any criticism or shame. Be thankful for the amazing job that your body does in so many ways. Enjoy the feel of your skin, the contours of your body and the ability to stretch and move as you wash yourself. Breath in deeply, appreciating the perfume of the soap or gel. Focus on how your breathing keeps going twenty-four hours a day, every day of your life. Bring a sense of awe and curiosity to your body about what it does for you and allows you to do. Your body is so much more than its weight, size or composition. Have a sense of enjoyment in being in your own skin.

Managing cravings

Use your journal to list the foods you crave. If you eat compulsively and find it difficult to know which foods you crave most, begin now to be mindful of how you feel around foods. Watch your behaviour with curiosity. Watching your behaviour around food is not about beating yourself up or having mental battles with yourself, just observe yourself for now.

Do you automatically reach for a handful of chocolate bars when you are at the check-out in a supermarket or petrol station? Be aware of your thoughts and desires. If you do feel a sense of criticism creep in, just say to yourself: *"Okay, I see I have a craving for another cake. I have had one already. I notice I have a powerful urge to eat another one. Is this what I really want?"* By pausing and considering your feelings and desires, the craving may pass. If it doesn't, see this experience as providing information to help you on your journey towards more peaceful eating. Ask yourself, what has the experience taught you?

Get help.

If you are struggling with BED, get professional help. A big aspect of BED is the shame and secrecy surrounding the binges. You do not have to be alone.

If you don't identify with all the aspects of BED but are frustrated by your compulsion to overeat, practice the suggestions in this book and share your experiences with others. Perhaps a trusted friend or family member would support you. Be at peace with yourself, your body and food.

The whole thrust of this book is to help you attain a sense of peace with who you are, the size you are and your behaviour around food. After years or decades of feeling fearful, alone, ashamed and disgusted, you can have hope.

Accept who you are for today. You only have today, so make the most of every precious moment. By constantly beating ourselves up or obsessing about food and diets, you are missing out on life itself. I sincerely hope that this book can help you regain your sense of peace and joy in life.

5. Meditation, Body, Scans, Movement and Breathing

Meditation practice isn't about trying to throw ourselves away and become something else. It's about befriending who we are already. Pema Chödrön.

Meditation

In this book I include guided meditations; one meditation for each week and an additional short meditation to listen to before a meal. There are also meditations in case you feel a binge coming on or have just had a binge.

Try just sitting observing your thoughts and feelings. This can be challenging and off-putting for inexperienced meditators. It can be discouraging to feel that you are constantly battling with your thoughts. Therefore, I encourage the use of the guided meditations to give you something to focus on.

It is perfectly natural to have lots of thoughts. That is how our minds work. By focusing on a voice, your body and breath you are directing your mind away from thinking to explore a stillness and space available to you but needs some training to make it easier. It is very difficult to sit in silence with no thoughts. I want to reassure you about this as I have seen so many people try meditation in this way, only to be bothered and discouraged by the endless stream of thoughts that bombard them. That is why I suggest the guided meditation to begin with. They give your busy mind something to focus on. You cannot 'just empty your mind of thoughts'. Please accept this and carry on with the guided meditations that are there to support you.

The Body Scan

A body scan is a structured mindfulness practice to help get in tune with your bodily sensations. Often we rush through life with little awareness of tension building up. It is only when we get back, neck or shoulder pain that we realize we have been holding tension in these areas. It is easier to prevent the tension from building up. The tricky bit is remembering to stop and take a moment to be aware of how we are feeling. The body scan helps with building this awareness that hopefully will become habitual.

Tension and stress can lead to a binge. By being aware of the tension building up, you take appropriate action. You might need to move, stretch, take a break, or change position.

The body scan will also help you tune into your sensations of thirst, hunger and satiety. Disordered eating will have disrupted these feelings.

The insula is the part of the brain that is responsible for interoception. Interoception is sensing what you feel inside your body. By tuning into your body regularly you are using the insula and interoception. Brain scans have shown that the insula gets bigger with more use. So keep practising the body scans and it will get easier to detect hunger, fullness and the build-up of stress.

Practising the body scan with self-compassion and gratitude for your body will help you feel more comfortable in your own skin. You will get more of a sense of appreciating yourself from the inside out rather than focussing only on your external appearance.

If you notice harsh judgement creeping in or a sense of discomfort about your body, just observe these reactions. Try not to let yourself be emotionally affected by your own inner critic. Remember, these are just thoughts; they only have power over you, if you allow it.

How to do a body scan

You can sit in a chair, lie on the floor, or sit on the floor as you wish. You must be comfortable. In time, with practice, you can do a body scan practically anywhere so you will need to adjust your chosen position to what is appropriate for that situation.

If sitting in a chair, ensure your feet are flat on the floor and that your back is upright and supported but comfortable and that your shoulders are relaxed and down away from your ears. Your lower arms and hands can be supported by the armrests of an armchair, or if you are sitting in a chair without arms rests, you can rest your hands in your lap.

If lying down, ensure that your back is flat on the floor, if you have lower back issues you could try putting a small rolled-up towel under your lower back where there is a natural gap between the floor and your back. You can lie with your legs stretched out on the floor, leaving some space between your legs and gently allowing the feet to turn out. If this is uncomfortable for your back, you can bend the knees and have the feet rest flat on the floor. If lying on the floor, ensure you are warm and not lying in a draught. The body scan is not a test of endurance but will hopefully be something to look forward to and enjoy as the time for some true self-care. Ensure that you are lying on a mat or thick rug and use blankets and cushions as needed to feel supported and comfortable. Make any adjustments you need to before you begin.

I appreciate that focussing on the body might bring up disturbing feelings or distracting thoughts. No need to struggle with these or try to resist them. Just notice them and try not to attach emotion to the thoughts. If you feel resistance or aversion, just observe this with an attitude of curiosity. Be compassionate towards yourself and your body.

Try to do one body scan every day this week as a minimum.

Script for the body scan guided meditation

The Body Scan

Find a place to sit or lie down comfortably. You can sit upright in a chair or lie on a mat or bed. If your thoughts wander bring them back to the body and the bodily sensations you are experiencing right now.

Bring attitudes of compassion and acceptance to this practice. If you feel any aversion or resistance to focussing on the body, notice this and try not to get too attached to the thought. Just let it go.

Bring your attention to the forehead. Close your eyes if this is comfortable for you, relax the jaw. Bring the attention to the throat and the back of the neck. Notice any tension you might feel.

Focus on the left shoulder, the left arm, hand and fingers. Imagine any tension or stress flowing down over your left arm and out through your fingers. Now bring your attention to your right shoulder and the right arm. Again, notice any tension you might feel. Imagine this moving down through the arm and out of the fingers.

Now focus on the heart area, keep your attention on this area, breathing in and expanding the whole chest cavity and down into the abdomen, allowing the diaphragm to drop and make more space for the lungs to expand. Notice any tightness around the ribcage. Stay with the breath in this area for a few moments. If you lose focus bring your attention back to the breath and the body.

Next, bring your attention to the stomach area, breathing fully into the stomach allowing the entire chest and abdomen area to inflate fully. Enjoy the sensation of fullness in the belly. Be thankful for the life-giving air your belly is holding for you. Accept its roundness and fullness. When you breathe out, just let the breath trickle out slowly and gradually with no force.

Now bring your focus to the back area, the upper back, the middle back and the lower back. Have a sense of how your whole back feels. If you are aware of any tension breathe into it and as you breathe out let the tension go, softening the muscles in the back.

Now focus on the area around the hips. Notice the sensations of sitting or lying. Be aware of the contact your seat area makes with the chair or floor. Notice any tension, breathe into it and let it go.

Bring your attention to your left thigh, the left knee, back of the knee, calf and shin. Have an awareness of the whole left leg. Now bring your awareness to the right thigh, the right knee, back of the knee, calf and shin.

Shift your focus to the left foot, front of the foot, heel, sole and ball of the foot; be aware of any sensations or lack of sensations in the toes. Feel how the foot rests on the floor. If barefoot feel how the air moves around the foot. Now bring your attention to the right foot, front of the foot, heel, sole and ball of the foot. Be aware of how the toes feel or be aware of any lack of feeling in the toes.

Have a sense of being grounded, a sensation of heaviness. Focus on an awareness of the solidity of your body. Breathe in deeply and slowly and notice any internal sensations in the body.

Feel any slight movement of air around the body or parts of the body. Be aware of the entire body.

If you notice any aversion or resistance to focussing on the body, just let it be. Notice it but avoid struggling with the thoughts or judging them.

After a few moments, bring your attention back to the room, you are in. With your eyes still closed, imagine the room in your mind's eye. Be aware of any sounds in the room or close to the room. Open your eyes stretch slowly and move on with your day.

A Note on 'Grounding'

As the book progresses, I will refer to 'grounding'. This means feeling our presence as a physical being on this earth. Be aware of the feet on the floor or ground. Take a slow breath in through the nose and have a sense of solidity and weight.

If you struggle with thinking of your physical weight, be aware of this, just notice it. Take a breath in and as you breathe out, let go of the fear and anxiety around weight. Assert your right to take up space in the world. Enjoy the physicality of your body and look on your feelings of solidity more in terms of a sense of security and presence.

When assailed by food cravings or the urge to binge eat we can feel out of control or deeply anxious. Grounding can give us a few moments to re-set and gain a sense of control and connect with a calm inner core.

By feeling your feet, perhaps planting them firmly on the ground and breathing well, we can give ourselves a feeling of security and support within our own body. You could say: 'Feel your feet' to yourself as a cue to be present in your own body and avoid the disconcerting light-headedness that can accompany stressful thoughts. You could also try walking around more slowly and deliberately, planting each foot purposefully on the ground. Just slowing down and being more intentional with how you move can interrupt the cycle of anxious thoughts about food or losing control.

Breathing

Focus on remembering to breathe through the nose, slowly and deeply. Breathe right the way down into the belly. If you struggle to accept the size, softness or roundness of your belly, just accept these thoughts and feelings and carry on breathing well. In our western culture, there is an emphasis on holding the belly in. This restricts full breathing and can lead to feelings of anxiety and fatigue.

These feelings can lead us to binge. If your body is fully oxygenated you will be less likely to feel tired or lacking in energy. If you do feel suddenly low in energy, don't reach for a sugary snack, pause and breathe well and then consider how you feel.

Movement

I use the word 'movement' and not 'exercise' deliberately. In our modern western culture, we push ourselves to exercise to counteract the effects of our sedentary lifestyles.

At this early stage, think about your attitude towards exercise or movement. Do you over-exercise to compensate for food binges? Do you dread moving around? Do you associate moving your body with punishing workouts or boot camp regimes?

It has been shown that moving our bodies gently at regular intervals during the day, every day is more beneficial than a strenuous workout at the gym for one hour at the end of a day spent sitting down. A study in the Netherlands in 2013 (1) showed that participants who were sedentary for long periods each day but did one hour of intensive exercise had less positive benefits compared to those who moved more during the day but didn't break out into a sweat. The lower intensity participants had better responses in terms of improved insulin sensitivity, a result that could lower their risk of developing Type 2 Diabetes.

It is much more beneficial, therefore, to aim to build gentle movement in during the day.

At this stage, as well as being aware of how you feel about movement, consider any movement you enjoy. Write a few ideas in your journal. Reflect on what you genuinely enjoy, not on what you think you should like.

Here are a few ideas to get you started:

- Walking–alone, with a dog or in a group
- Dancing
- Stretching
- Pilates
- Cycling
- Jogging
- Gardening
- Running around the park with your children
- Cycling
- Rollerblading
- Water-based sports such as surfing or sailing
- Team sports such as netball, football or cricket
- Golf
- Tennis

Don't overlook good old-fashioned activities like giving the house a deep clean or sorting out the garage; anything that gets you moving, if it is a sociable activity, such as dancing, a class or team-based activity, even better. You will be busy making friends, moving naturally and with enjoyment. Food will be downsized to its rightful place as a source of nutrition and just one aspect of life that gives pleasure, amongst a range of activities.

As you are engaged with the activity, pause at points to consider how you are feeling, physically, mentally and emotionally. Look around you and fully experience the moment with all of your senses. Remember to breathe well, breathing through the nose and inflating the belly.

Do activities you enjoy and give you pleasure. As you are engaged with them, be mindful of the benefits you feel as you are involved with them.

If you do feel mild discomfort during physical activity, this can be of benefit to reset our behaviour around food. Usually, feelings such as anger, anxiety or fatigue are resisted. We turn to food to change these feelings as quickly as possible. By experiencing some slight discomfort, we can build resilience and tolerance and experience the feeling, knowing it will pass, without having to turn to food to immediately change it.

Please note, I am referring to mild, minimal discomfort. Please do not push yourself into the threshold of pain. Forget about 'no pain, no gain' – exercise is not punishment.

I am talking about just being on the edge of comfort. This is the proximity of growth and progress. We treat our bodies with compassion and respect, but we can still move to strengthen muscles and build endurance.

Start small, be consistent, and move often.

6. Mindful Eating

Over the next few weeks, I will encourage you to practise mindful eating. This means that when you are eating, you are fully present to the experience. I have included a short, mindful meditation to listen to before each meal.

I appreciate that it might not be possible for you to listen to this before every meal. You may eat lunch at work and it is not practical for you to listen to a meditation in this environment. However, I would urge you to listen to the meditation before at least one meal a day. For the other meals, I would ask you to at least pause before eating. Perhaps take a moment to feel or express gratitude for the food on your plate. You could reflect on all the hard work it has taken to produce the food and get it onto your plate. Take a few deep breaths into the belly and notice how you feel.

Before you eat, ask yourself if you are hungry. This hunger scale might help you pinpoint whether you are hungry: Get into the habit of regularly checking in with yourself to check on your hunger rating.

1. Starving–feeling shaky and weak.
2. Very hungry–low energy, growling stomach feeling tetchy.
3. Quite hungry–stomach making some gentle growling noises.
4. Starting to feel hungry.
5. Okay–neither hungry nor full.
6. Satisfied and contented, feeling pleasantly full.

7. Feeling a bit too full. Stomach feels slightly stretched.
8. Feeling over-full/stuffed.
9. The stomach is aching.
10. Feel sick and too full.

Feel the sensations of hunger–a feeling of an empty stomach and intestine area, a dip in energy, a rumbling stomach. Have a glass of water and ask yourself if you still feel hungry. Hunger can be confused with thirst. Do not restrict food, but you want to get in touch with your body. Binge eating can disrupt physical cues to eat. If we have been eating to comfort and soothe our emotions, we get disengaged from the physical aspect of genuine hunger.

Mindful eating is also about engaging all of our senses in the experience. Before you put any food in your mouth, appreciate the colours of the food. Notice any contrasting colours such as bright red tomatoes with sprinkles of vibrant green herbs. Breathe in the food's aroma with appreciation and anticipation.

As you eat, be aware of the texture of the food in your mouth. Is it chewy or soft? Are you craving a certain texture? Chew slowly, fully experiencing the flavours and textures of the food.

Put your fork down between bites. Take your time to enjoy the meal. Try to make the meal last for twenty minutes. This gives the body time to register that food has been ingested. Eat until you feel comfortably full, but not overfull. Enjoy a sensation of satiation balanced with a comfortable sense of lightness. You do not want to feel overfull or stuffed. This helps retrain the body and mind, moving away from the urge to stuff food in until the stomach feels stretched.

Enjoy the meal and savour all the tastes, textures and aromas as you eat. Notice how you feel physically and emotionally. Has your mood changed as you have eaten? Are you aware of any cravings? Do you have any fear or anxiety around the food you are eating? Do you fear a loss of control or overeating? Are you comfortable with the sensation of fullness in the belly? Take a moment to appreciate the body and how it can extract the nutrition it requires from the food you have eaten.

This might seem a lot to remember. Practice what you can. The following acronym might help to prompt you:

PEACE.

Pause – before beginning to eat.

Enjoy – savour every mouthful.

Assess – assess your levels of fullness as you eat.

Chew – chew slowly and thoroughly.

Enough – when you have enough, finish your meal.

Take your time and appreciate the meal. Try not to rush your food. Use all of your senses and enjoy.

Before Meals Meditation

This is a short meditation to complete before meals. When you have listened to it a few times, you will go through the process yourself drawing no unwanted attention from others. Try to eat at a table with minimal distractions.

When you sit down to eat. Look at the food on your plate. Take a moment to do this. Breathe in the food's aroma. Anticipate the taste and texture of the food in your mouth. Close your eyes for a few seconds and be grateful for the food. Consider all the hard work and effort that has gone into producing the food and cooking the meal.

Open your eyes and pick up your cutlery slowly. Enjoy your meal, giving it your complete attention.

7. Summary

We have covered a lot this week. Well done for sticking with it. I have introduced many key concepts that we will refer to as we go through the next few weeks. I hope that you feel that you have a solid foundation from which to move forward.

If you have missed out on the reading for any of the days this week, catch up today.

I have emphasised that this is not a diet book. Let go of any restrictive thinking and focus on health and well-being in a holistic sense that is physical, mental and emotional.

I have introduced a good deal of mindfulness practices this week: meditation, the body scan, breathing, mindful eating, and a focus on pleasurable movement.

This book can be of help to anyone who struggles with overeating or binging, no matter what end of the spectrum they are on.

I have asked you to do some practical things to help support you. If you have not looked in your cupboards or had time to clear out your wardrobe, don't worry. Perhaps find some time today? There will be other opportunities to do this, but the sooner you can clean up your environment, the easier it will be to find peace and contentment with food and with yourself.

I have given you some tips to deal with urges to binge. These are just to help you through these first days and weeks. The strategies in the rest of the book will help you in the long term.

Above all, I hope you have been clear about what is motivating you to practice mindfulness. This clarity will help keep you on track as you move forwards over the next few weeks. Record your hopes, wishes and dreams but don't get too caught up in the exact outcomes. Let's move forward on this journey with a sense of curiosity and openness. Let life unfold.

A reminder of the daily actions:

1. Read the daily section, reading one section each day.

2. Listen to the guided meditation for the week once a day. (See Appendix 1 for instructions on how to download your audios.) If you can also listen to the short meditation before a meal, that would be wonderful.

3. Take five minutes each day to record your thoughts in your journal.

Week Two

Cravings, Binges and Triggers

To thine own self be true. **William Shakespeare**.

As Maria ate the cake, she felt a sense of relief. She relished the sensuous texture of the cream, chocolate, and sweet and icing. A feeling of relaxation washed over her as she sank her teeth into the velvet texture of the birthday cake. Her stomach rumbled, and she responded with an urgent gulping of more cake, chewing and swallowing quickly. The sweetness was intoxicating. Maria felt as if she could never stop. She brought to mind the round figure she saw in the mirror. She was unhappy with how she looked, but the urge to indulge was too great. She pushed large handfuls of the soft cake into her mouth, cramming it in. Tears streamed down her face as she realised she couldn't stop…

Meditation for Dealing with Cravings.

Today we will reflect on meeting our genuine needs and how to let passing cravings go. It is important to meet our physical and emotional needs promptly. Instead of chasing our desires and ignoring our needs, we will focus on learning to attend to what our bodies and emotions need to thrive and stay well.

A craving could be for something your body needs, so honour your cravings. Notice them and make a decision that is good for you. We are not setting strict rules or restricting. However, if you have a craving that you know will lead to a full-scale binge, you will want to observe the craving but let it go. By ensuring you meet your needs and have a nourishing diet, you will be less likely to have troubling cravings.

Now, take a few moments to get comfortable. Make any necessary adjustments and settle back into the chair or the mat. Be aware of the points of contact your body makes with the surface supporting you.

Take a deep breath in through the nose and breathe out slowly. Consciously release any tension as you breathe out. Watch the breath for a few moments.

Focus now on your body. If any distracting thoughts come to mind about your body. Bring your attention back to my voice and let the thoughts go. Imagine a torch is shining on each area as you move up the body, showing up any tension or tightness. As I name various body parts, take a moment to experience how that area feels now. Begin with the feet, then the legs, the knees, the thighs, the hips, the abdomen, the chest, the back, the shoulders, the arms, the neck and the head. Bring your attention now to the area around the heart.

Put your right hand over your heart and consider your emotions today. Accept the first word that comes to mind describing your feelings in this moment. On the next out-breath, drop your hand.

Think back over an average day. Reflect on how you usually meet your needs. Do you leave adequate time to cook and enjoy nutritious meals? Do you get enough sleep and rest? Do you make sure you are hydrated? Do you seek company if you feel alone? How do you comfort yourself if you feel low?

Commit to meeting your needs promptly in your daily life. Resolve to meet your genuine needs and let unhealthy cravings go. Focus on self-love and self-worth. Make choices that support your self-esteem.

Now bring to mind a mental picture of yourself engaged in an activity that you find absorbing. Feel the feelings you have when you are engaged in this passion. Focus on the feelings of pleasure and intense interest. In your daily life whenever a craving hits you, bring to mind this mental picture and make time for this activity.

Be mindful of what you really need and turn your attention to making a healthy choice that re-affirms your self-esteem and self-worth. Bring to mind anything you feel you need right now. You may need something physical, like a drink of water or to move. You might have an emotional need such as some connection with another human being in the form of a hug, a chat or a smile. As we come to the end of this meditation, commit to meeting that need when we finish. If you have nothing come to mind, enjoy these few moments of peace and freedom.

Now, take a stretch and carry on with your day.

Additional Meditation to Overcome an Urge To Binge, or Recover From A Binge.

Settle yourself as comfortably as you can. You may experience intense tension and agitation. Watch your breath. Is it fast and shallow? Deepen the breath and breathe more slowly. Be aware of your heart rate, can you feel your heart fluttering in your chest? Put your right hand on your heart and feel it beating, as you slow your breathing you may notice the heart rate starting to settle. However, it is for you today, observe the heartbeat. Continue breathing in slowly for a few minutes. You may wish to close your eyes to help focus on the internal sensations.

With your hand still on your heart, commit to accepting yourself just as you are now. Be aware of any intense feelings or emotions. Accept the emotion. Observe the effect it has on your body. Remind yourself that these feelings will pass. Breathe in deeply and as you breathe out allow the powerful emotions to move through you like the wind through a tree. See the emotion as energy being shift as you breathe out deeply. Let your hand drop.

Now bring your attention to your jaw. Relax the jaw and the face. Be aware of any tension in the shoulders, do a few gentle circles with the shoulders and breathe out deeply, letting any tension go.

As your agitation settles, ask yourself what you need right now. Take a few moments to consider this.

Commit to taking some action to meet your needs when you finish this meditation.

Take as much time as you need to sit quietly and breathe well, enjoying these few moments of peace. When you are ready, move on with your routine; ensure you take some action to nurture yourself and treat your body with respect and gratitude.

1. The Reality of Food Addiction

Until recently, food addiction was considered a myth by most health professionals. For some, the jury is still out. However, with brain imaging and further research, it is now increasingly accepted as an authentic form of addiction.

Without getting too tangled up in research that proves or dis-proves food addiction, it's worth noting that people don't usually overeat kale, apples or broccoli.

Many people shy away from food addiction, sensing the stigma around addiction: perhaps associating addiction, only with drugs or alcohol. However, addiction is no reflection of someone's moral fibre or character; it is just a physiological phenomenon. Some people might be more prone to addiction than others because of a complex mixture of brain chemistry, life experiences and learned habits. Although some people might be more pre-disposed to addiction whether it's food, alcohol, drugs, social media, gaming, gambling, risk-taking, exercise or sex, all of us have the propensity to get addicted to something in our lives.

If you struggle with acceptance around your body size or your behaviour around food, perhaps finding out more about how certain types of food can be addictive, might help. You are not weak-willed or a failure. You may have been at the mercy of an addiction. This might help you be more compassionate with yourself. Equipped with the knowledge of food addiction, we can then adjust our behaviour around food, to make choices right for us as individuals mindfully and compassionately. This is not an excuse to give up, as we can be in control of our behaviour and actions around food. We might just need to be more aware of our habits and reactions to food.

Certain types of food, especially combinations of sugar, fat, and salt has been shown to trigger the reward centres in the brain. The same centres triggered by substances such as cocaine. It would seem that like most addictions, some people are more predisposed to food addiction than others. The causes can be a complex mix of genetic factors, life experiences, and personal emotional and physical factors.

The biochemical process underpinning sugar addiction can be explained in four steps:

Step 1. After we ingest sugar, the increase in blood sugar forces the pancreas to secrete insulin. As the insulin breaks down the sugar, blood sugar levels will drop.

Step 2. When blood sugar levels drop, a signal is sent to the brain, telling it blood sugar levels need to rise.

Step 3. The brain releases hormones that cause cravings for sugar. The person feels weak and mildly agitated.

Step 4. The sugar addict will then binge on sugary food to satisfy the craving.

There has been debate around whether food addiction is literally to the food or to the eating behaviour. Let's look at the example of eating cake. If we habitually eat huge portions of cake, we could be physically addicted to the 'high' this highly palatable food gives us. Or we could be addicted to the behaviour - that is eating the cake at a certain time in certain conditions. If we eat cake when we get home and we do this every day, we could just be addicted to the behaviour.

By being mindful of our eating patterns, we can disentangle the complex set of motivations and behaviours that have slowly built up. You can practise mindfulness around the problem eating by asking yourself the following questions and noting the answers in your journal:

- How do I feel before I eat this food? Note your physical and emotional state?
- How do I hope to feel after I have eaten this food?
- How do I feel if I attempt to deny or resist the urge to eat this food?
- Can I choose not to eat it, or do I feel an overwhelming compulsion to eat it?
- Is there another way I could meet my physical or emotional needs rather than eat this food?

In his book *The Pleasure Trap*. (1), Dr Doug Lisle refers to 'magic foods'. These foods are highly palatable and usually contain extensive amounts of sugar, fat and salt. They are the foods that we just can't help going back for more of. They have been deliberately manufactured to have us craving more. Food scientists manipulate the exact amounts of salt, sugar and fat to reach a 'bliss point'. Food companies want to sell more food to keep their shareholders happy. It's not a conspiracy, it's just business, but we need not be victims. However, it might feel like they catch us in a cruel trap.

I remember once working with a client who desperately wanted to stop overeating foods such as biscuits, cakes, and pies as his health was being badly affected. He also felt a damaging loss of self-esteem, shame, and a sense of being out of control around food. He cried as he told me how he had binged on a full packet of biscuits, even though he didn't want to eat them due to his fears around his health.

What was happening here was that the highly palatable food was overriding his rational mind. His 'thinking brain' wanted to avoid the food, but the more primitive part of the brain, which is activated by the combination of refined flour, fat, and sugar in the biscuits, was too powerful. These overwhelming urges combined with the stress response, triggered by anxiety caused by our conflict around the food, can just be too much.

You are not weak-willed or lacking in some mysterious moral strength, it just means that your brain circuits are working in the way they were intended to work. We are hard-wired to seek high-calorie foods, going back to our ancient ancestors. If this wasn't the case, humanity might not have survived. In ancient times, refined sugar and flour did not exist in the form or volume it does today. Rich foods, such as honey or nuts, were only found occasionally and the effort to get them was intensive. Think about the need to brave bees to get to the honey, or cracking open nuts without nutcrackers. Getting these rich foods took much effort, and consequently, they were eaten in moderation.

Food addiction is not the same as Binge Eating Disorder. Food addiction may affect this disorder, but for people suffering from BED dealing with self-esteem and deep-seated emotions are significant issues. I will address these in Weeks 4 and 5.

Today, if you are still binging, overeating compulsively, or struggling around a certain food, just notice your feelings with compassion and curiosity. Be kind to yourself and acknowledge that you might be in the grip of addiction.

Your mindfulness practice will help you navigate a personal route through food choices to come up with a pattern of eating which will nourish and be peaceful for you.

Signs of Food Addiction:

- Overwhelming cravings.
- Eating more than you want to eat.
- Feeling guilty about what you have eaten.
- Over-exercising to expend the calories consumed.
- Setting rules around food and then breaking the self-imposed rules.

- Hiding food and eating alone.

Today we have taken a brief look at food addiction. The scientists are divided, but anecdotally we know that we are more likely to over-eat ice cream than lettuce.

You have experienced the overwhelming pull of certain types of food. By being present with your eating and behaviour, you can pinpoint the foods and situations problematic for you and take some mindful action. This could be not keeping problem foods in the house or making plans for alternative activities when you know you are vulnerable to over-eating.

For example, coming home from work is often a time when people over-eat. You could have a small snack before leaving work, to ensure you are not physically hungry and go for a walk or do a dance class after work before you go home. By doing something pleasurable to de-stress from the day, you may be less tempted to binge on comfort foods when you get home. The first step is being present and aware. Make some notes in your journal of what you have noticed about foods you crave. What strategies have you tried? What has worked?

If you have time today, if you have not done it already, I would encourage you to write a compassionate letter to yourself to read in the event of a binge. Imagine you are comforting a dear friend; write all the nurturing things you would say to your friend to comfort them. Be supportive and reassuring.

If you have binged this week, please be gentle with yourself. Let go of that 'all or nothing' thinking. Just because you have had a slip, or a binge does not mean all is lost.

I hope you have listened to the meditation today.

2. Nourishment for Body and Soul

Perhaps in the past, you have tried to gain some control around food by imposing strict rules and restricting what you eat. You might have skipped meals and struggled with genuine hunger and low blood sugar levels. You might have tried very restrictive diets or followed an eating plan that only allowed drab frozen ready meals in disappointingly small portions.

This sense of deprivation and lack can only go on for so long. Your list of what you could not eat seemed so much longer than the list of foods you were allowed to eat. No wonder you weakened and splurged on the highly palatable food. Your brain's reward system had been trained to recognise these foods as the ones that would make you feel better. You were simply reacting to how you had been conditioned.

To underpin your mindfulness practice, you need to feel well physically. Food needs to:

1. Keep your blood sugar levels even.
2. Provide fibre and fluid to ensure you feel full.

3. Give your body macronutrients (carbohydrates, proteins and fats) and micronutrients (vitamins and minerals.)

Switch your mindset to one of looking to food for nourishment. I understand that some of you might be worried about weight gain. The thought of not being on a diet might make you feel like you will just be out of control. However, by eating nourishing food regularly throughout the day your body will learn to trust that it will get what it needs. You will come into balance and cravings will diminish.

In each meal seek a balance of vegetables or fruit, carbohydrates, protein and healthy fats. Unprocessed foods such as vegetables, beans, fruit, whole grains, lean meat, fish, tofu, and greens will help keep you full and satisfied for longer, stabilise blood sugar levels and provide your body with the fibre and nutrition it needs. These foods are nutritionally dense, that means they have more of the vitamins and minerals your body needs.

When I talk about carbohydrates in your plan of eating, I mean wholefood, unrefined carbohydrates, such as brown rice, whole-wheat pasta, whole-wheat bread and starchy vegetables such as potatoes, turnips or parsnips. These are filling and nutritious. These foods release serotonin and make us feel satisfied. Fill up on these foods; unrefined carbohydrates are not the enemy.

Refined carbohydrates, such as white bread, biscuits or white rice can make blood sugar levels spike and the consequent fall in blood sugar can make you feel jittery and light-headed. This feeling could be the precursor to a binge. You want to aim to keep your blood sugar nice and steady. So fill up on unrefined carbohydrates.

Proteins help keep us satisfied for longer and help the body to repair. If you want to avoid meat or fish because of ethical reasons, there are plenty of plant-based proteins to choose from. Try a variety of foods. If you hate a food, don't force yourself to eat it. Eating a wide variety of food will mean you are getting the nutrition you need and will keep cravings at bay.

Enjoy your food but keep it in its rightful place as a source of nutrition and something to enjoy within a range of enjoyable experiences. Eating for fun occasionally is great. Enjoy it! But, using food as your only source of comfort or pleasure could be problematic.

We need to eat for balanced nutrition and sustenance and move away from constantly seeing food as our only source of entertainment and comfort. In the early stages of this mindfulness journey, I suggest that you take care with so-called 'trigger foods'. Trigger foods are usually highly palatable items very high in saturated fats, sugar, and salt, which can disrupt the body's natural mechanisms of hunger and satiety. Salty food can make us feel bloated and uncomfortable. You may feel that you are comfortable having these foods at home. If you are, trust yourself. If you feel unsettled, nervous or out of control around these types of foods you may want to free yourself of their temptation in the early days and weeks of your recovery.

This does not have to be a 'forever' situation. No food is banned.

Plan ahead

Shop mindfully; keeping in mind the principles we have talked about today. I usually buy a wide selection of fruits, vegetables, beans, pulses, cereals and have a well-stocked spice rack. I love to experiment with my own recipes and find that if I have plenty of fresh, wholesome food at home I can come up with lots of meals. Alternatively, you might enjoy looking up recipes and shopping for the ingredients. Do what works for you but I would encourage you to keep the following points in mind:

- Write a shopping list.
- Consider online shopping.
- Batch cook and freeze meals.
- Don't food-shop when you feel hungry.
- Stick to the outside perimeters of the shop where the fresh produce usually is displayed.
- Keep some 'emergency' meals and snacks at home for those times when you are too tired or busy to cook a nutritious meal.
- Keep some wholesome snacks handy in your day bag or office drawer.
- If you are busy or stuck for ideas try services such as 'Hello Fresh'. Fresh ingredients, herbs and spices are delivered to your door with a recipe to prepare a healthy meal.

Take a few moments to think about what would suit your lifestyle, pocket and tastes. By planning ahead and shopping mindfully you will be giving yourself the optimum chances of success to beat binging.

How much is enough?

I understand that your perception of how much you need to eat has got all out of whack. Each person will vary in their needs according to activity levels, size, gender, genetics, age and lifestyle. Eat regularly - three meals a day with two snacks. Don't go for more than three or four waking hours without eating. Avoid constant grazing. If you feel hungry between meals and it will be more than an hour to your next meal, have a snack. If you know you will eat a meal soon, experience mild hunger and enjoy your next meal.

Your stomach is roughly the size of your clenched fist, so aim for roughly this amount of food in each meal. There is useful advice on the UK NHS website on healthy eating (www.nhs.uk/live-well/eat-well/the-eatwell-guide). The NHS eat well guide recommends that we eat at least five portions of fruit and vegetables per day. A meal should consist of one-third fruit or vegetables, one-third carbohydrates and the rest of the plate made up of protein and dairy (or dairy alternatives) and a small amount of fat. Aim for a rough balance across the day, as it won't be possible to have these exact proportions at each meal. Don't stress over exact amounts, this is just a guide. If you overeat snacks, try having pre-portioned snacks such as mini bags of nuts or crackers or wholemeal biscuits in individual-sized wrappers. I love nuts and tend to get carried away eating from a large bag, so I pre-portion nuts into smaller bags or prep-boxes ready for snacks. This can help in the early days of adjusting to eating in moderation (but NOT restricting).

In your journal, record how you see your relationship with food today. Does it feel like a struggle? Do you have distinct trigger foods you do not yet feel safe around? Which foods feel nourishing to you? Do you need to make any practical adjustments to your shopping habits or meal preparation? Make a note of them in your journal.

Commit to eating regular, nourishing meals.

3. Are There 'Good foods' and 'Bad foods'?

There is a lot of confusion around food. Which is the best eating style? However, we are all individuals. Ideally, the foods you choose to eat are based on your tastes, ethical considerations, levels of activity, age, build genes, height, sex, location, and even the season.

No one eating style fits all people. Instead, focus mindfully on your preferences and what feels nourishing and safe for you. Eating foods that make you feel good in the longer term. If you lose control with ice-cream and end up feeling sick and unwell, this is a self-defeating and unkind act towards yourself. Re-educate yourself to be gentle and compassionate. Rather than beat yourself up, find an alternative activity to eating ice-cream. An activity that is nurturing and enjoyable. We will look at this mindfulness strategy in more detail next week on Day 4.

Many people say they overeat because they love food. The first few bites of a cake or chocolate are always the best. When we overeat, the food loses its taste. We begin to feel uncomfortable, both physically and emotionally. If we love food, then let's just focus on the first few bites and savour it. Practise doing this in a 'safe' environment for you. By that I mean eat foods you crave when they are more controlled, for example, buy one cake with your coffee if you go out with a friend or order one dessert, perhaps to share with your partner when out for a meal. If you know you will lose control with that family-sized tub of ice cream, when at home on your own, then avoid this situation.

You may have a history of diets and restrictive eating, designating some foods as 'bad' and others as 'good'. This thinking is too binary. No doubt there are foods that you don't feel you have control around. Or foods that make you feel unwell.

As we have seen, certain foods are highly palatable and trigger brain chemicals such as dopamine. The chemical composition of these foods drives you to eat more and more, losing any sense of satiety or fullness until you feel over-stuffed and nauseous. These are usually highly processed foods with a list of strange-sounding ingredients that sound like the elements of a science experiment. In his book *The Pleasure Trap* (1).Dr. Doug Lisle refers to these foods as 'magic food'. This 'magic food' is designed to get us to eat more and more of it. Food scientists call the addictive perfect balance of fat, sugar, and salt the 'bliss point'. Sadly, this 'bliss' is short-lived and becomes ever more elusive as you eat more and more to experiences the pleasure once gained from these highly palatable foods. Like any other drug, tolerance levels build and it takes more and more of the substance to get the same feelings.

This is a very personal reaction. You need to work out for yourself the foods that rob you of peace or control. By being mindful of how you feel around a range of foods you can work out which foods are safe for you to have in your environment and which foods you feel you lack control over. This does not make any food good or bad per se.

Rather than considering foods as 'good' or 'bad', it is more helpful to think of foods as your 'staples' (those being the foods that form the bulk of what you eat on a day-to-day basis) and 'occasional foods' (those being foods that are highly palatable, less nutritionally dense and more energy-dense, such as cakes, sweets and crisps). This way you have a nutritious and filling basic diet with a few add-ins for fun and variety. No need to deprive yourself.

Try following an eating plan that includes a range of unprocessed whole foods, one that includes proteins, natural fats, unrefined carbohydrates, and lots of fruits and vegetables. It will take some time to adapt to foods free from all the additives, sugar, processed fats, and salt, present in the 'magic foods' that are causing you problems.

Look on these 'staples' such as fruit, vegetables, beans, and brown rice as foods that you can be at peace around. They are filling and nutritious. You can eat them until you feel satisfied with no guilt or shame. As you adjust to what might be a new of eating for you, be mindful of how you feel. Give space to any feelings of resistance or non-acceptance. You can notice them and move on. Consider how food is cooked and seasoned. Have a little salt or sugar sprinkled on a meal if this makes nutritious food more palatable for you. Have a bowl of porridge with a sprinkle of sugar, rather than a box of doughnuts.

If you have been starving and then binging on refined foods such as cakes and biscuits, there will be a period of readjustment. This process of adjustment is called neuroadaptation. This is when we are re-training our brains and taste buds to enjoy unfamiliar food. In time, the reward centres of the brain will re-set and will respond as nature intended to whole, unprocessed foods with feelings of satisfaction and pleasure.

Earlier in the book, I asked you to let go of all or nothing thinking. If you eat in a way that is nourishing and healthy, you have not wrecked your health by eating one cake or a dessert. As you establish a pattern of regular eating of satiating and nourishing food, you will be less tempted to gorge on high fat, high-sugar foods. You will regain more trust in your ability to control yourself. If you have one cake, that's fine.

I hope you can listen to the guided meditation today. Remember to make some notes in your journal today; perhaps reflecting on the foods you consider 'good' or 'bad'. Ask yourself, do you have an 'all or nothing' attitude towards food?

4. Life's Abundance.

Life is so much more than food, diets, and exercise regimes. Food is a basic and pleasant aspect of life, but let's put food into perspective. Meal planning, shopping, working out what food we enjoy, what food helps our bodies to function well, eating socially, enjoying a treat, all these activities can be enjoyable. However, obsessing about food, hoarding it, feeling frightened by food, feeling out of control, punishing ourselves because we have eaten or hurting our bodies to get thin is life-sapping and depressing. Find peace with food and eating. Find out for yourself the foods that work best for you and put food in its rightful place as a part of living a full and vibrant life.

In the section on self-care, we will look at different aspects of taking care of ourselves. For now, write a list of things you enjoy doing. This could be anything from reading a novel to watching the sunset or taking your dog for a walk. Life is rich with experiences; don't confine yourself to the fridge and the sofa.

Build up your cornucopia of enjoyable activities that enhance your life and make you feel good.

When trying out a new activity or returning to something you used to enjoy, do so with a mindful approach. Consider how you feel before, during, and after the activity. Do you look forward to it? Do you feel excited? You might feel nervous, don't let this put you off. How quickly does the time go by when you are involved in the activity? Afterwards, do you feel uplifted, inspired, or just happy to have been involved?

We have also talked about the mindfulness attitude of compassion. Be compassionate with yourself. Forgive yourself for any slips or mistakes as you make efforts to change your binge eating patterns. It will take time and patience.

Have fun

Mindfulness is not all about sitting cross-legged on a gluten-free meditation cushion looking serious. You are allowed to feel joy and have fun! Think about all the things you used to enjoy as a child. Flying a kite? Going for a bike ride? Making a scrapbook? Growing a plant from seed? Make a note in your journal of some things you enjoyed doing and make time to do them soon.

Connect with others

Binge eating can be a lonely and isolating experience. Reach out to others; get involved in your community. When you meet up with friends or family practise listening mindfully; giving the person your full attention, not interrupting, not being concerned about what you should say back or give advice, just be present for that person. The bonds and sense of belonging you will form with others will help ease the fear, loneliness, and isolation binge eating has brought into your life.

Be grateful

Cultivate a sense of gratitude for the people you have spent time with during your activities. Be grateful for your ability to get to the location or venue for your activity and for the time you have to do it. If you feel that you did not enjoy the activity, be grateful for the information you now have to make another choice.

Celebrate

Take the time to reflect on all your efforts, no matter how small. It takes courage to try unfamiliar things and meet unknown people. Well done.

Use your journal to make a list of activities you have enjoyed in the past, or that you think you might enjoy doing. Tomorrow, we will look at how you can make these ideas more intentional.

5. Automatic pilot

Automatic pilot is the technology that keeps an aircraft on course without the intervention of the pilot. It refers to those occasions when we fulfil actions without thinking or being fully aware of what we are doing.

You may have had the experience of driving on a day off or a weekend, only to take the route to work. You had not intended to go to your workplace, but you realise part-way through the journey you are following your usual daily route. This is automatic pilot, it is unthinking behaviour. Your feet and hands are moving to control the pedals and move the gears, but your mind is elsewhere.

Automatic pilot starts as a useful adaptation for learning. Imagine if we had to re-learn routine behaviours every day? How inconvenient it would be is we had to think about how to get out of bed, how to put one foot in front of the other to walk, how to brush our teeth and so on. We can learn habits so well that our brains register nothing new or out of the ordinary, so we can perform tasks without even thinking about them. We become 'habituated'.

You might think this habituation is a helpful thing because of how tedious and time-consuming it would be to have to re-learn mundane tasks every day. Learning a skill, whether it is how to walk, ride a bicycle, play the piano, drive a car, or operate machinery is all helpful.

The problems arise when the habits become so automatic that we proceed without thought or attention to the task in hand. When anything happens, that is unusual while we are cruising along on automatic pilot, we react rather than respond. Perhaps you have reached out for food and eating it without thinking. When you get upset has it become automatic for you to overeat?

I remember once visiting a close friend who struggled with eating behaviour. As she chatted and bemoaned the state of her health, in particular her weight, she had eaten an entire tray of biscuits. When I pointed this out to her, she was genuinely shocked and found it difficult to believe she had eaten so much in one sitting.

Your habitual reaction to food might be to eat it. By realising this is automatic pilot and using mindfulness techniques to break out of it, you will respond to food rather than automatically reacting to it.

Reacting and responding are different. When we give a response in any situation, it is by definition responsive; it is thoughtful, measured, and considered by our rational selves as appropriate to a situation. However, when we react, it is usually a quick, thoughtless, automatic reaction that may have undesired consequences. Consider this scenario:

Maria arrived home from work, late. She felt tired and rattled after a busy day in the surgery. She had picked up her sons from the childminders and they were playing happily in the garden. Maria's mind drifted off to a conversation she had with one of the GPs that day. He had talked about cut-backs because of lack of funding. Maria sighed and opened the biscuit barrel, taking out a chocolate biscuit. She started munching on a biscuit as she pulled out plates and crockery to set the table for dinner. She continued to eat one biscuit after another as she moved about the kitchen, her mind partly on the meal preparation and partly on the conversation at work. She put her hand back in the biscuit barrel and was surprised to see it was empty.

Maria has just munched her way through a packet of biscuits on automatic pilot. How often does this happen to you?

By learning to be present in the moment you are breaking the habit of automatic pilot. By taking a few breaths, pausing and asking yourself how you are in any moment, you are more able to respond rather than react.

In the above example, Maria was distracted by her thoughts about the day; she was also busy preparing dinner and was just acting out of habit, the habit of walking into the kitchen and eating on the go. If Maria focused on the task and let the thoughts from the day go, she would be more present. Maria did not want to eat so many biscuits before dinner, but her unthinking mind took over and she acted out of ingrained habit.

By pausing and asking ourselves if our behaviour–is in line with our intentions and goals, we create a brief space to make more considered choices. We might ask ourselves if we are hungry. If the answer is 'yes' you will then eat as a response to the hunger rather than reacting on automatic pilot. If you are not hungry or you are preparing a healthy meal and know you will eat soon, you can then choose not to eat.

Spending our lives in automatic pilot means we miss out on a lot of joy.

6. Have a Plan

In Week 3 we will look at the mindfulness attitude of acceptance. Acceptance is not about passive resignation about a situation. Acceptance is an active choice. Today accept yourself as you are with an understanding and compassion for your struggles. This week we have looked at how food addiction can control your choices and behaviour around food. I hope this has helped you to let go of any shame with a lack of control around certain foods. No wonder you eat too much of some foods, they have been designed that way.

However, you can change the behaviour that is causing you pain, interfering with relationships, and possibly affecting your health and sense of well-being.

When I refer to a plan, I am not focusing on goals. I am focussed on habits that will support you in making the changes you want to make. I am interested in lasting behaviour change that will have an impact and benefit in your life.

You will form your own eating plan based on some broad principles laid out this week and on any medical or health needs you may have. It will form part of a plan of recovery. It is important to consult with your doctor about the foods and levels of exercise right for you, especially if you have BED or any other health challenges.

The plans will look different for each person. Everyone will start at a unique point. The following are some headings to think about. Write your plan in your journal and refer to it daily as part of your routine. Change it and update it regularly to celebrate your ongoing achievements and success. If you go off-plan, just readjust and pick up where you left off.

No beating yourself up, you are letting go of shame and criticism.

Headings for your plan:

- How I can keep my environment diet free?
- How I can nurture a positive body image?
- How I can adopt an individual eating plan (with your health professional if required)?
- How I can deal with cravings?
- How I can build in mindfulness practices daily?

- How I can include activities that make me feel good?
- How I can connect with others?

The following is an example of how a plan might look. I have based this example on the needs of Maria. You remember that we have been learning about Maria's struggles each week so far.

Maria's plan:

- How I can keep my environment diet free?
  Clear out all my diet books. Throw out the diet shakes. Do it this on Saturday morning.

- How I can nurture a positive body image?
  Go clothes shopping and buy clothes that fit me now. Give away the clothes that don't fit. Do this on Saturday afternoon.

- How I can adopt an individual eating plan?
  Shop on-line once a week. Get a veg box delivered. Eat four meals a day. Don't skip meals. Eat at the table with Sam and the boys. Have healthy snacks ready for when I get home from work.

- How I can deal with cravings?
  Eat all my meals and avoid getting over-hungry. Ask Sam to keep his snacks and treats out of sight. Have fruit available and in sight for us to snack on as a family. Have dessert on Sundays when I have time to savour it. When cravings hit and I am not

hungry, I will leave the kitchen and look at Pinterest for a few minutes. I am planning a holiday in France and am enjoying pinning pictures of places I would like to visit.

- How I can build in mindfulness practices daily?
  Listen to a guided meditation each morning. Pick on attitude per day and practice it that day. Write in my journal at bedtime, noting three things I am grateful for. Eat lunch away from my desk, mindfully.

- How I can include activities that make me feel good?
  Go clothes shopping with my friend Amy, who I can confide in.
  Go to the park with Sam and the boys on Sunday. Write in my journal. Plan a weekend away with Sam.

- How I can connect with others?
  Practice compassion with colleagues at work. Use the time at the dinner table each evening to talk and listen to Sam and the boys. Switch off the TV and spend time with Sam in the evenings. Go out with Amy, who always makes me laugh.

This plan will work in harmony with the practical steps outlines earlier this week on how to eat in a way that nourishes your body.

Make the plan your own. Every individual is different, so a one size fits all plan will not work for everyone. This is a plan to help get you started on the path of a peaceful relationship with food and your body.

7. Summary

This week we have looked at the concept of food addiction. We have seen how some foods are potentially more addictive than others because of the chemical composition of the food. I hope that this knowledge about food addiction helps you to view your difficulties with more self-compassion and understanding. You are not weak or morally defective.

By clearing out your cupboards of your trigger foods; you will set yourself up to make life easier and more peaceful in these early weeks. This does not have to be forever. The more effort you have to put in to get food that triggers a binge, the more chances you have of success to stick to your desired eating plan. This feeling of success will have a positive effect on your self-esteem and feelings of mastery over food.

Emotions will impact profoundly on your eating. We have looked briefly, at how emotions affect your eating behaviour. If you did not get time to complete the Traffic Light exercise last week, do it today. Keep this exercise in mind as you go about our day and check in with your emotions and urges to eat.

Did you have time to write your letters to yourself? One letter to help remind you of all the reasons you want to stop binging and another to comfort you if a binge has occurred. If you didn't get time to write the letters, take some time today.

I hope you have more of a sense of food as being just part of an entire range of pleasurable experiences in life and that you will try some new activity this week and see how it feels.

Yesterday I urged you to make a plan to support you as you go forward. If you did not have time to complete the plan, revisit that section and make a plan to help you on your mindfulness journey towards peace with food.

This week I Have also urged you to use your journal to record the following:

- List the foods you crave most often – consider how you will manage these foods – will you have a total clear-out or keep them at home in small portions? The choice is yours, but do what will give you the most peace of mind.
- List the strategies you feel have worked best in helping you overcome cravings.
- List any new activities you would like to try or activities that you would like to make time for in your life, which you used to enjoy.
- Make a list of appealing activities to get busy with if a binge urge descends on you.

If you didn't get time to complete any of these journal entries this week, spend a few moments now making noting your thoughts. This will help clarify your thinking, and also by recording your thoughts, you will commit these strategies to memory. This commitment to memory will serve you well next time you feel you are in a troublesome situation around food.

Listen to the guided meditation and use the time to re-read any sections from this week you feel you would like to revisit.

Over the next few weeks, we will delve deep into self-esteem, emotions and body image issues. You can use your journal to make notes on any of these issues. Remember, you can use your journal as a mindfulness tool, to pour out your feelings and raise your awareness of your thoughts, habits and patterns of behaviour.

Week Three

Attitudes of Mindfulness

We cannot force the development of mindfulness. **Allan
Lokos**.

Maria woke up, groggily aware that it was the early
hours. The streetlight streamed through the window.
She sighed and turned over, trying to get into a comfortable
position. She felt hunger gnawing, reminding her of her
earlier self-denial, skipping the birthday treat meal she had
prepared for everyone else. Maria turned onto her back and
sighed. She felt wide awake.

After a few moments, Maria's mind turned back to the
afternoon. She smiled at the memory of the children's
laughter and games. As a child, Maria had never had a
birthday party, not a proper birthday party with friends,
games, sweet treats and a cake with candles. She suddenly
felt tearful. Maria sat up in bed, checking quickly that Sam
was still asleep before she slipped her feet into her slippers
and crept out of the bedroom quietly.

As Maria descended the stairs, she caught sight of herself
in the mirror on the landing. Despite her efforts to avoid all
the treats, in her eyes, she looked dumpy and fat. Her mind
drifted back again to the party that afternoon. All the other
mums there had looked slim and trendy in jeans or light
summer dresses. She had dressed in a baggy black
tracksuit. Maria had a wardrobe full of clothes she could no

longer fit into. She sat at the top of the stairs and felt tears well up. She was trying so hard, but nothing seemed to make a difference.

If she could just get some sleep, she would feel better tomorrow. On automatic pilot, Maria carried on going downstairs. She walked into the kitchen and put the kettle on. As she waited for the water to boil, she caught sight of a reflection of herself in the kitchen window. She felt a wave of revulsion wash over her. Maria opened the fridge and reached for the cake leftover from Joe's party

Meditation on Attitudes of Mindfulness

Sit or lie down. Settle into a comfortable position with a straight spine. Close your eyes. Bring your attention to your breath. Allow the breath to flow freely without changing the breath or trying to control it. Let the breath come and go. Notice the rise and fall of the abdomen as you breathe in and breathe out. On the next out-breath let the shoulders drop a little and enjoy a sense of release in the shoulders. Let this feeling of relaxation move down the arms. Be aware of a sensation of heaviness in the hands. Bring the attention to the feet and feel the weight of the feet. Bring the feeling of relaxation up the legs and into the area around the hips. Deepen the breath a little and bring the attention back to the abdomen and chest. Observe again the rise and fall of the chest and abdomen. Sit for a few moments watching the breath.

Thoughts will probably come. Accept this, but resolve not to attach any emotion to the thoughts. On the next out-breath let the thought go. See it as 'just a thought'. Take in

a fresh breath and enjoy the stillness. Again, if a thought enters your mind, just let it go on the next out-breath.

Now, listen to these words, remaining silent as you listen and focusing on your internal reactions to each word: compassion, letting go, non-striving, gratitude, acceptance, patience, non-judging, willingness.

Now, choose an attitude to focus on in your meditation today.

You might choose the first word that comes to mind or it might be an attitude you feel you would like to cultivate in yourself.

Consider your feelings about this attitude. Notice any sensations that come up for you. Accept your feelings.

Bring to mind any situation you would like to bring this attitude to. This could be a relationship or a situation at work or home. Spend a few moments reflecting on how you could practise your chosen attitude in the context you are meditating on.

Now spend a few moments reflecting on what has come up for you. If you feel neutral, accept this and enjoy sitting quietly for a few moments, keeping your focus on the breath.

On the next in-breath, deepen the breath and on the out-breath open your eyes and stretch. Now carry on with your day.

1. Compassion

By being more compassionate with ourselves, we free ourselves from the self-loathing and the harsh inner critic that can drive us to binge eating.

Acceptance of ourselves and our situation is the key to begin the process of change. If we are constantly at war with our bodies, our appetites and our life situation, we are constantly in a place of angst and discomfort. We will often turn to food to seek the comfort we crave. By letting go of the struggle we can feel more at ease and comfortable, thus avoiding the need to seek external comfort in the form of food.

Avoiding harsh self-judgment is part of the process of acceptance and of instilling habits of compassion. We will improve and get better with gentle nurturing and encouragement, not by constantly beating ourselves up.

In developing these attitudes and by incorporating new mindfulness habits and responses in our lives, we will need to let go of some old patterns of thought and behaviour.

Last week I asked you to be mindful of the triggers for your binges. Continue the effort to be consciously aware of when, how, where, and what type of food triggers binges for you. Bring these attitudes of mindfulness to these efforts.

If you are still binging, be compassionate with yourself. This means avoiding listening to the inner critic. Have a growth mind-set; instead of thinking; *"I can't believe I've done it again. I am a (insert insult here)..."* A growth mind-set response would be *"I have binged on ice cream. I feel uncomfortable and disappointed. What can I learn from this? I was looking for comfort. If I feel I need comfort, I will choose something to do that I enjoy such as a warm bath. I missed lunch today, so no wonder I was hungry! I will make sure I eat lunch from now on."* This constructive self-talk helps us to feel more positive and hopeful as we move forward.

Compassion–connection, not perfection.

Compassion reminds us of the deep bond we have with others. Einstein referred to this when he talked about the self-imposed prisons of thinking we are separate. He urged people to: 'Widen our circle of compassion to embrace all living things.' Be compassionate with yourself and others. This will help in the following ways:

- Your self-esteem will go up.
- By being compassionate, you will develop and be aware of personal attributes that are nothing to do with appearance or weight.
- It will shift your attention and focus out towards others and away from the internal struggles you have had with food and body image issues.
- You feel connected with others, breaking the isolation felt by many binger eaters.
- You will feel more emotionally fulfilled and happy by being of service to others.

Being compassionate is a process, not just a feeling: The first step of the process is to be present.

Be present in your own life; experience fully what is going on in any one moment. You will have heard the phrase 'be present' before, but what does 'being present' mean? Feel the sensations in your body. This might be a challenge for you. You might avoid tuning in to how your body feels because the harsh inner critic steps in with many judgements. Use the body scan technique to tune into how your body is feeling. Accept what comes up for you and see it as just information. Replace the inner critic with the inner nurturer. Don't argue with the critic, look at it without emotion attached and foster compassion and acceptance.

The other aspect of being present is being aware of your thoughts. Many people are bothered by thoughts when meditating, but mindfulness is seeing the thoughts, being aware of the thoughts coming and going but not get caught up in the thoughts.

By being present, we are also aware of our emotional experience at any moment. We will talk more about emotions later in the book, but it is a helpful practice to pause and ask ourselves what we are feeling emotionally in that moment.

So being present means being aware of your feelings, thoughts and experiences

We can be present for other people by listening with an open heart and mind. This means we accept them as they are. We avoid being distracted by phones or emails while with the other person. We give them our full attention.

The next stage of compassion is being in-tune with the other person, feeling empathy and human identification. Compassion for others will help us feel better about ourselves, our lives, and to build better connections with others. This sense of connection will end the dreadful sense of being alone and isolated.

The last stage of the process of compassion is wishing the best for that person or intending to relieve their suffering. This can be a practical action, or if we cannot take a practical step, we could make a sincere wish that their suffering is alleviated. You can also apply this to yourself. Wish the best for yourself. Take positive action. You are doing this now, by reading this book and following the suggestions.

The following are some ideas of how you can practise compassion towards others:

- Small acts of kindnesses: in the form of courtesies to strangers when driving or moving about.
- Helping someone you can see is struggling.
- Phoning someone just to ask how their day has been.
- Sending a note or card of appreciation.
- Making someone a hot drink.
- Avoiding retaliating when irritated with someone.
- Being patient with an elderly or infirm person.
- Allowing yourself and others to make mistakes.
- Accepting that human beings are not perfect–that includes you.
- Accepting situations as they unfold.

- Practising loving-kindness meditations or repeating to yourself the following:

May I be happy.

May I be safe.

May I be healthy, peaceful, and strong.

May you be happy.

May you be safe.

May you be healthy, peaceful, and strong.

Binge eating is usually a secretive and lonely activity, separating us from others, cloaked in shame and feelings of self-loathing. By actively fostering a more compassionate attitude in our lives, we are building bonds with others to overcome loneliness and isolation. By being more compassionate with ourselves, we are building the foundations for a kinder, more loving, and healthy relationship with ourselves and our bodies. By having compassion for our struggles and feelings, we will find more nourishing and sustaining ways to meet our needs. We will stop beating ourselves up with food.

By being compassionate with others, we are creating bonds that help us break out of the prison of disordered eating and shame.

I hope that you will listen to the guided meditation today and make an entry in your journal on what might come up for you as you reflect on the attitude of compassion.

2. Acceptance

Acceptance is an *active process* of choosing to accept what is going on in the present moment. We don't have to like it or force ourselves to enjoy it.

By accepting ourselves just as we are, we can forge a healthier, more respectful relationship with ourselves and our bodies. We need not be at war with cravings, or the bathroom scales, or with food. By accepting situations as they are, we can get more comfortable with who we are and where we are in our lives. We can make plans to live more healthfully. We can forge new habits and responses to difficult life experiences. We can change and grow and move on, however, we need not fight or struggle to do it. The first step is to accept how things are now.

Make space to allow for whatever situation or experience it is. We can plan to remove ourselves from the self-destructive habit of binge eating. By accepting our feelings as they are without denying them, we can free ourselves up from the reflex response of stuffing the feelings down with food. We need not negate, ignore, or deny our feelings. We can accept them, experience them, process them, learn from them, and move on.

Acceptance does not mean we have to stay stuck in a situation that is causing us pain. But, by accepting your feelings around the situation, you can make changes.

We are all susceptible to the effects of modern advertising. The beauty and weight loss industry will tell us we have a problem; we are too fat, too old or the wrong shape and the list could go on. The advertisers hook onto our insecurities. They point out the problem and they can provide the solution. They manipulate us into an attitude of non-acceptance. Our appearance is unacceptable. Our weight is unacceptable or our lines or grey hairs are unacceptable. So bringing acceptance into our lives is an active process and goes against habitual ways of thinking.

Just play about with this attitude; imagine how it would feel to accept yourself as you are in this moment. You might have hopes and dreams of feeling more at peace with yourself and food, acceptance can be part of attaining that peace you desire. We are so accustomed to attacking projects head-on; that it can be difficult to believe that by accepting something we can access the peace we crave.

Remember, acceptance is not resignation. You can take positive action. Taking positive action is better than staying stuck in negative action such as feeling or acting angry, fearful, and frustrated or, depressed. When we accept the present moment we invite fresh energy into a situation, a lighter energy of hope, possibility, and choice.

I hope that you will listen to the guided meditation today and make an entry in your journal on what might come up for you as you reflect on the attitude of acceptance. This might involve acceptance of your body, your thoughts and emotions or acceptance around the history of your behaviours with food. You can choose new behaviours, but by practising acceptance of what has happened in the past you are freeing up the emotional energy to enjoy the present and move forward with hope.

3. Non-judging

When I talk about judging I mean the harsh judgement that has undertones of negative criticism, blame, and shame. We can use our discretion and intelligence to judge that a situation or person may not be safe for us.

We can use our intellect to give useful feedback on a piece of work or a project to help improve it or extend skills. Genuine feedback will be specific and will be balanced with some positive comments. Harsh, generalised or off-hand 'feedback' is not usually helpful. This condemning judgement lacks any authentic desire to assist the other person to improve or extend their skills. If you are the recipient of this judgement, try to take something constructive from it, if you can, and then let it go and move on.

In relating to others, non-judging is part of acceptance and compassion. If we are with someone we accept them just as they are at that moment. We don't get hung up on what we don't like or focus on aspects of their personality or appearance you think they should change.

You are present with them, in the here and now, just as they are. This includes you.

Today, be aware of how often you fall into the habit of judging yourself. Perhaps you do it when you see yourself in a mirror or when you make a slight mistake or speak up in a group. This constant judgment invokes the inner critic and sets the scene for comparison with others.

If we could free ourselves up from the fear of our own or other people's judgments, think how free you could be to be whom and what you are truly meant to be. Fear of other people's poor opinions of us can paralyse us; it limits growth and creative endeavour. It is perfectly reasonable to ask for and accept feedback, but unsolicited opinions are the business of other people. Stay in the centre of your own life and don't get too caught up in the judgments of others.

Yesterday, we talked about how the beauty and fitness industry can encourage us to not accept ourselves. The advertisers urge us to judge ourselves harshly. They present air-brushed, computer-manipulated images of perfection that no real human being could compare with. This constant self-judgement and comparison have become endemic. By getting into a space of acceptance and non-judging, you are overturning a lifetime of habitual thought patterns. These thoughts might be conscious or just a low background sensation of being inferior in some way. By consciously nurturing a non-judgmental attitude, you are making room for acceptance of whom and what you are.

Be aware of your own 'inner critic' and don't get caught up in your harsh self-judgments–see them as just 'thoughts' and let them go.

If you are in a relationship with someone who is judging you harshly, pay attention to what is going on. Set some boundaries and remind them you are taking action to feel better. Explain that harsh criticism hurts you and is not helpful. Speak up for yourself. Later in the book, we will talk about people-pleasing. We do not have to accept unreasonable behaviour from anyone, hurtful judgemental comments are abusive.

As you listen to the meditation today, be aware of what comes up for you when you think about being non-judgemental. Make a few notes in your journal or think of areas in your life in which you feel judged either by other people or your inner critic.

4. Letting go

Powerful emotions such as fear, anxiety, resentment, and anger can set off a binge. Irrationally, we may stuff in the food in anger and resentment, as if that will get at the other person. By practising more healthful ways of dealing with these emotions, such as letting go, we can avoid some triggers for a binge.

One mind-set I would ask you to let go of is seeing everything in a binary system of good and bad, right and wrong, feast or famine. This thinking can lead to a binge. If you eat one chocolate biscuit, you need not eat the whole packet. This thinking may have come from strict diets. You eat one sweet, so you've broken the diet so you might as well eat the entire bag. One biscuit or one sweet will not make a lot of difference. Let go of this 'all or nothing' way of thinking about foods or 'forbidden foods.'

Practising tolerance, acceptance, and compassion with a situation that evokes anger, fear or resentment can help. Taking the person or situation out of your head and into your heart might work.

In practical terms, that means letting the angry/worried/fearful/resentful thoughts go. Instead of ruminating on past injustices/fears/what-ifs/what might have been and so on, focus on your heart and channel the emotional energy of the situation away from the head and into the heart.

In this way, you are acknowledging how important this situation is or has been to you. You are not dismissing it; you are redirecting it to a place where you will be less mentally bothered by it.

Also, trusting your heart with this person or situation will soften the harshness, disappointment, judgment, or anger that might surround the situation. Above all, accept that letting go is a process. Sometimes it's a lengthy process. This is not usually a once and for all dramatic occurrence.

In particular, you may experience troubling anxiety about food. You might worry about an upcoming social event that revolves around food, or a holiday season that involves feasting on foods you crave. By fully experiencing the anxiety, looking at it, sitting with it and accepting it for what it is–a feeling, you can then let it go. You can then be free to make choices that are not motivated by fear or anxiety.

We can find that we let one thing go, and then something else pops up. That's being human. Keep working on letting go as a continual work in progress. There will be much more about dealing with emotions later in the book. Besides letting go of troubling emotions, we may need to consider letting go of:

- Obsessing about diets and weight loss.
- Trying to please others, to make ourselves feel better.
- Patterns of behaviour that do not serve us.
- Unrealistic expectations of appearance.
- Certain food that triggers cravings.
- Places or situations that trigger over-eating behaviour.
- People who put you down or judge you.
- Books, social media sites, magazines, products or objects that trigger feelings of inadequacy or imperfection.
- Punishing fitness regimes.
- Uncomfortable or ill-fitting clothing
- Instant gratification. Get more comfortable waiting to have a desire fulfilled. This slight discomfort will train your mind to recognise that all cravings need not be instantly satisfied. You could practise this with many things, not just food, for example, impulse clothes shopping. If you see an item of clothing you want, put it on a wish-list and wait.

Make a list of anything you feel you need to let go of. If you need to let go of some material objects, do it today or make a note in your journal of when you will do it. Be alert to any other inner prompts of things you might need to let go of as the days and weeks go on. As you listen to the guided meditation today, be open to any thoughts or feelings regarding letting go that might come up for you.

5. Gratitude

Gratitude can be a game-changer. By being aware of all the pleasurable things in our lives, we take the power away from food as seeming to be the only way we can find comfort or joy. When we are reminded that we are surrounded by many wonderful experiences, people, and material blessings, it takes the focus off food.

Gratitude increases our sense of happiness and enjoyment of life. By consciously being aware of all the varied things in life we are grateful for, it takes the emphasis off food as our only comfort and solace. It also increases feelings of joy and connection with others. Having a sense of gratitude for the people, experiences, material resources, natural phenomena, interests, and hobbies help us see life in a more balanced way. Happiness is not at the bottom of the biscuit barrel. You can discover it all around you every day.

By being grateful for the miracle of your body and mind, you will be more inclined to treat your body with the respect and nurturing it deserves. You won't want to overwhelm your system with massive amounts of fatty, sugary foods.

Be grateful for your food. Eat mindfully and appreciate every mouthful. This will help you slow down your eating and enjoy your food healthily and naturally.

Be present, appreciate what you sense all around you, and be grateful. By filling our hearts and minds with thoughts of gratitude and appreciation, we are filling up mental and emotional space that could be filled with negativity, fear, anxiety, and resentment.

First, just notice what you are grateful for. What do you value and appreciate in life?

- Your spouse.
- Your family.
- Your friends.
- Your home.
- A walk with the dog.
- An enjoyable book.
- A sunny day.
- A comfortable bed.

In your journal, write at least three things you are grateful for every day.

By practising gratitude for what you have around you, you can transfer this attitude towards your body. You don't have to think your body is perfect or beautiful to be worthy of gratitude. When practising gratitude for your body you could focus on:

- Your bodily processes and functions, heartbeat, breathing and digestion.
- Your senses being able to see, hear, touch, taste and smell.
- How your body helps you enjoy activities such as singing, running, walking or dancing.
- Communication–talking, listening and expressing your feelings and opinions.

You could open a file on your computer where you write what you are grateful for and keep adding to the list. When you feel low or feel that you will turn to food for comfort, open up the file and read about all the things you are grateful for.

You could keep a jar at home with slips of paper, on a slip of paper, write something you are grateful for, and put it into the jar.

You could do this with your family and share memories to be grateful for. This will help you by lifting your mood, being present with your loved ones, and being a grateful role model for your children. This is a sustaining and nourishing activity to complete with your family.

In your journal, write three things about yourself that you are grateful for. Add to this list as you go forward; practise being grateful for yourself. As you listen to the guided meditation, reflect on what gratitude means to you.

6. Willingness and Trust

Be willing to change and see your life situation and who you really are in a fresh light.

Be willing to let go of old habits and routines that you are weary of. It might feel frightening to let go of the crutch of food. It might feel like food is your only friend and that you are letting go of something that is familiar. For now, just be willing to consider letting these learned responses go. Be willing to try out some new responses and form some healthy habits to cope with the challenges of life.

Be willing to try out the attitudes discussed this week. If an attitude feels difficult to practise; write about this difficulty, dig deep to see why this might be. The insight might give you that 'aha' moment that can help you understand and change perspective.

You need not do everything I have suggested so far in the book but be willing to try out a few of the techniques or ideas I present.

Trust

You may have lost trust in your ability to recognise hunger. You may have lost trust in your ability to control yourself around certain foods. You may have undergone some trauma or loss and lost trust in life itself.

Gently, try to allow a sense of trust in your life. I understand that this might be frightening. You may have put your trust in diets, diet plans, weight loss coaches or slimming clubs and feel they have let you down. The beauty industry has swindled you into trusting them to make you feel attractive.

As we have said before, feeling vibrant and enjoying life is an inside job. No one, no product or number on a scale can make you feel attractive. The euphoria of attaining a certain weight won't last. It is time to trust yourself. If you make genuine, small, daily efforts to treat yourself and others with compassion, gratitude and acceptance, you will most likely feel more at peace with yourself and the world. Bit by bit, your ability to do what is right for you and to trust your instincts will return. Be patient.

Use your journal today to write about your feelings regarding the attitudes discussed this week. Which ones are easy for you? Which of the attitudes to you feel any aversion to? Which areas in your life do you feel you need to use more willingness towards – letting go of certain behaviours or items? Treating yourself with compassion? These are just a few ideas to get you thinking.

7. Summary

As the quotation at the beginning of this week says, we cannot force the development of mindfulness; however, by keeping these attitudes in mind day to day, you will perceive a gradual shift in perspective.

Fostering a sense of compassion, acceptance and gratitude for yourself will help develop respect for your body and your emotional needs.

I intend the guided meditation to provide some space in which to reflect on these attitudes and your feelings about them. These insights can help you be aware of the blocks that could hold you back.

The following are some questions to reflect on:

- Have I challenged my inner critic?
- Have I responded to it with compassion for myself?
- Have I expressed gratitude for my body?
- Have I resolved to let go of old patterns of reacting to difficulties or uncomfortable feelings?

You may want to re-read a section on an attitude covered this week or use some time to clear out anything you have let go of. Record any feelings, observations or insights you have had this week in your journal.

Well done on completing the third week of this book. Your commitment deserves recognition and respect.

Week Four

Emotions

Nothing ever goes away until it has taught us what we need to know. **Pema Chödrön.**

The children ran around the garden as Maria looked on, smiling. "Penny for your thoughts? "Sam asked, looking quizzical. "You looked miles away. I just wondered what you were thinking." Maria shrugged, "Oh, I was just thinking how happy they all look. I'm so pleased they are all having such a lovely time'' Maria gave Sam a bright grin. She realised her mind had drifted back to her own childhood. She had never had a birthday party. Not a proper birthday party with friends and games and cake. Her mother didn't enjoy having 'strangers' in the house. The house was an embarrassment, anyway. Maria felt shame at the thoughts of it all. Her mother was a virtual recluse, trying to keep Maria at home for as long as possible. Her mother would warn her of all the awful things that could happen if she left home. She would lament on at length about how people could not be trusted and eventually, everyone lets you down. Maria had only found the strength to leave home when she had met Sam. She had trusted no one else, and she was eternally amazed that he was interested in her. When Maria told her mother that she and Sam were getting married her mother fixed her with a sour look and said: "It won't last." Maria was fearful that perhaps her mother would be right.

Meditation on Emotions

You can sit upright in a relaxed position or lie back on a bed or mat. Settle comfortably but keep your spine straight. You can close the eyes or keep them open, but allow the gaze to be soft and unfocused. Keep your jaw relaxed and be aware of the feel of your tongue against the roof of your mouth and behind your teeth. Allow for some space between your upper and lower sets of teeth.

Gradually bring your attention to the breath. Notice if it is shallow or deep. Are you breathing into the upper chest area or the abdomen? Is the breath fast or slow? Notice the air coming into the nose–does it feel cool. As the breath leaves the nose, how does that feel?

Notice your emotional state today. Name it quickly and let the thought go. No need to analyse it just now. If you feel in a neutral state, be aware of this. Sit quietly for a few moments, observing what comes into your mind and the effect your thoughts have on you.

Notice how internal events such as memories, bodily sensations, or particular thoughts can influence feelings and emotions. Reflect on how external events or conditions can influence thoughts and emotions.

Bring your attention back to the breath. Breathe deeply into the abdomen and keep your focus on the abdomen. Fully experience the inflation and deflation of the belly. As you breathe in, focus on the word 'peace' and as you breathe out, focus on the word 'calm'. Continue to breathe in on 'peace' and out on 'calm' for a few moments.

Sit now for a few more moments, reflecting on the words 'peace' and 'calm'. If you feel any agitation or disturbance, bring your attention back to the breath, and as you breathe out allow a small sigh to escape, releasing the tension.

Have a sense of openness and space in the body. Breathe in, fully inflating the ribcage, let the breath go. Experience the movement of the breath through the body. Make room for your emotions to flow through the body. See your emotions as an energy that can move through the body and be released. No need to hold on to emotions or push them down. Experience the emotions; be aware of all the bodily sensations that indicate a certain emotion and use the breath to let the emotion be released.

If a difficult emotion comes up, use the breath to help ease the intensity. Use words such as 'peace' and 'calm to soothe yourself and help you sit more comfortably with any distressing thoughts or feelings.

Make space for what you feel right here and now and accept your emotions as they are today. Reflect on how they will change. Focus on fully experiencing them now, as they are.

On the next out-breath, begin to move the head. Tuck the chin in towards the chest and then look up towards the ceiling. Look over the left shoulder, then over the right shoulder. Roll the shoulders back and then forward. Focus on a detail you can hear in the room or close by and bring your attention to your immediate external environment.

Slowly stand up, perhaps stretch gently and carry on with your routine.

1. Emotional Eating

Is emotional eating the same as binge eating? Not necessarily. Everyone indulges in emotional eating sometimes. Many of us enjoy cake at birthday celebrations, attaching the idea and enjoyment of cake with the joyful nature of the occasion. On a chilly winter's evening, a bowl of warm soup or stew can give us a sense of comfort. You might associate a particular meal with a certain ritual or habit you have formed in your family or as a couple. So we are all emotional eaters.

However, emotional eating can become a problem if it is the *only* way that you deal with emotions. By using food as a constant crutch or means of celebration, you are at risk of running into health problems. Emotional eaters rarely go for broccoli or apples. It is usually food that can set off a pattern of addiction such as high fat or high-sugar foods.

Emotional eaters can be male or female. We can give children unhelpful messages about emotions as they grow up. As a teacher working with young children, I would see first-hand how very little boys would talk about 'loving' their friends, male and female. They would be affectionate and open with their feelings. At around age seven to eight, this seems to change. Boys want to seem tough and strong. They learn to hide emotion and learn to use jokes and banter and avoid discussing feelings. Boys and men may use food to cope with this lack of an emotional outlet.

By using food as the only way you deal with emotions, you are neglecting more healthful ways of managing emotions. For example, if you have an argument with your spouse and you walk away, going straight to the fast-food drive-through to stuff down your feelings, this will not help you sort out the issues that caused the argument. It also means you are not processing the emotions that have come up for you. Perhaps you are angry with your spouse but are too frightened to express the anger as you fear a break-up. This is obviously not an effective way to deal with any issues in your relationship. This can become a pattern across all your relationships that can cause problems for you as an individual and harm the quality of those relationships.

So-called 'good' feelings can bring on an emotional eating splurge–the euphoria of a party or joyful event can open the floodgates for excessive eating too. If this is occasional and linked to a social event, it probably is nothing to worry about, but if it is regular, secretive and causing distress, it needs to be addressed.

It is natural to take pleasure in food, but that pleasure needs to be in the right proportion with all the other pleasures available in life. If food is the only pleasure and becomes the single go-to substance to deal with emotions, we need to take stock and be mindful of the role food plays in our lives.

Remember, we can't fix emotional hunger with food. When you overeat to handle an intense emotion, ask yourself what are you truly hungry for? What do your heart and soul yearn for? In week one I urged you to record in your journal your hopes, wishes and dreams. Have a look back at what you wrote; this may give you an insight into what you really crave.

Shaming yourself, restricting or using willpower to stop binging will not work in the long term. In Week 2 I listed some tips to help deal with cravings, but these are just first-aid measures to use in the short term. To deal with the causes, we need to work through our emotions. These emotions could be very intense. Mindfulness can help by fully experiencing the emotion but being aware we are not the emotion. For example, if I feel anger; I can be curious about my anger. I can ask myself questions about it. In doing so, I can get some answers and process the anger without feeling overwhelmed by the feeling. I am not the anger I am just experiencing the emotion of anger. The emotion is a signal for me to ask a question and take action if necessary.

To illustrate this point, I once worked with a client who I will call Claire. Claire lived alone; she was the youngest of four sisters. Their father was dead and their mother was in a nursing home. Sadly, Claire's mother had Alzheimer's and her health was deteriorating rapidly. Claire felt overwhelmed by sadness because of her mother's condition. She found that she had established a habit of going to bed early to watch TV in bed. She would eat vast numbers of chocolate bars while she watched TV and cried. She felt disgusted at herself and was distressed by the amount of weight she had put on in a short space of time.

Claire was an emotional eater. She needed help in identifying her emotions, accepting them and processing them without constantly using food. I encouraged Claire to talk about her family life growing up with her mother, father and sisters in a small town in Ireland. She spoke about her father's alcoholism and how his rages terrified her mother and sisters. Claire was frightened to express her own powerful emotions and used food to stuff powerful feelings down. Her mother and sisters didn't discuss their father's behaviour. Feeling to do so would be disloyal and critical. After his death at forty-five, the sisters never talked about their father or their experiences growing up. I encouraged Claire to talk to her sisters about their childhood experiences and feelings about their parents.

Claire's eldest sister refused to discuss any of these issues, but Claire could talk to her two middle sisters about their memories and feelings. This was a lengthy process, and Claire had additional help; the sisters attended a 12 step programme for the adult children of alcoholics. Over time, Claire lost interest in binging on chocolate at night. She felt connected and close to her sisters and felt she had an outlet for intense emotions. This illustrates the point; the binging was not about the food. Claire did not need to use willpower or short term fixes for cravings because she worked through the emotions of fear, anger and shame from her childhood. Her heart needed the connection with her sisters. This deeper bond has helped them deal with the pain and sadness of their mother's illness.

As we come to the end of today's section, please be clear that emotions themselves are not the problem. Avoiding or pushing emotions away with food has become the problem. Perhaps the emotions have just felt too overwhelming. Issues with food often start in the teenage years – a time of great emotional upheaval. Patterns of using food to cope with emotional intensity are established and as an adult, it can be difficult to establish new habits. By using mindfulness practices you will be creating new responses to dealing with difficult emotions. You are not broken; you are human. Don't wait until you are emotionally 'fixed' to get well. Emotional experience is a lifelong process. It is part of the human condition to feel emotion – sometimes intense emotion. Mindfulness can help us to sit with emotions and not try to change them with food.

If you have experienced trauma or having severe difficulties with your emotions, please do get specialised help.

By sustaining ourselves physically (with nourishing food and movement) and emotionally (with self-care, compassion and acceptance), we will be less likely to use food to soothe painful emotions.

In your journal, make a note of how you usually deal with distressing emotions. Perhaps reflect on a recent off-day or argument with someone you care about – how did you deal with the emotions that came up? If food is your only way of dealing with intense emotions, a mindful approach can help you by:

1. Dealing with distressing feelings – observing, detaching, and being curious.

2. Provide a range of activities to practise self-care to help work through the uncomfortable emotions–guided meditation, a body scan, noticing your environment, recording your feelings in a journal. Absorbing yourself in an activity such as mindful movement or colouring.
3. Bringing to mind attitudes of mindfulness such as compassion, gratitude, or letting go. These attitudes can change our perspective and help work through difficult feelings.

Before closing this section today, it is also worth noting that our physiology can affect our emotions. We are biological beings. If you have been eating erratically or binging on sugary foods, they will affect your moods; a crash that can make us feel jittery will follow a blood sugar high.

Other factors might come into play, such as female hormonal cycles. I would encourage female readers to track your menstrual cycle and be mindful of your emotions over the month. The insights you get could help you plan ahead. The difficult feelings associated with Premenstrual Syndrome or Premenstrual Dysphoric Disorder (a more intense and distressing form of PMT), could then be more manageable. For example, you could ease up on work and social commitments at this time or make sure you are stocked up with non-food items that help you feel better. These could be books, magazines, baths oils, scented candles or a box set.

If you are experiencing dramatic swings in blood sugar levels, have a medical check-up to rule out any conditions such as hypoglycaemia or pre-diabetes.

It takes great courage to be open to powerful emotions. It might feel very intense, but I would urge you to stay with your efforts to experience your emotions, especially if they are painful. Reach out to others and get support.

In the words of Gábor Máté: 'The attempt to escape from pain is what creates more pain.' (1). The work that you are putting in now will help you in the long term. Use self-compassion and self-care to soothe you. Get help and support and don't struggle alone.

I hope you can listen to the guided meditation today and reflect on how changeable our emotions can be. Don't judge how you will feel tomorrow by how you feel today.

Use your journal to write about any feelings that may trouble you. Get support if the emotions are very intense. Talk to friends and family about your feelings. Make connections with others. These connections will sustain you and activate feel-good hormones; so the temptations of binging on your food of choice will lessen.

By identifying your emotions and letting them work through you, you will fill that 'hole in the soul' that you have been trying to fill with food.

2. Anger

Anger is a natural reaction to injustice whether for ourselves or on the behalf of others. Anger can give us the impetus and energy to make necessary changes. There is nothing wrong with feeling angry or in expressing anger appropriate to the situation. Looking someone in the eye and calmly expressing your feelings of anger about a situation can be powerful.

Often, people who binge eat are stuffing their anger down with mashed potatoes or cake. They may feel that they cannot express their anger. This might be for fear of the response or because of worries about being rejected. Anger turned inwards can turn into self-pity and depression and it will spill out, eventually. Often the anger erupts suddenly and shockingly, taking everyone by surprise.

People can stay stuck in a self-defeating loop of denial of anger, avoiding feeling it and confronting it. As well as food, people might use co-dependent relationships, shopping, or compulsive busy-ness.

Look back at your early childhood and think about how you expressed anger as a child. How did your parents, siblings, teachers, and friends react to your anger? How was anger expressed in your family? Are you aware of times when you actively suppressed your anger? How did this feel? During the time you are thinking about anger, be aware of your bodily sensations and feelings in the present. If you have an urge to eat, don't eat. Wait for thirty minutes while you consider your anger. Make some notes in your journal about what you remember from your childhood and how you feel about anger today.

If you are feeling angry about the denial of your feelings in the past, or about an issue from the past, feel the anger. Movement can help to shift the anger. Go for a brisk walk or a jog. Dig the garden or do some kickboxing. Have a sense of the anger coursing through your body. Feel its energy rushing out of your arms, into your hands, into your feet, and out of the top of your head. Let the anger go. If you feel sadness at how you were treated as a child, fully experience the sense of sadness, without eating. Cry if you need to and acknowledge the feelings. Let the sadness drain out of you with the tears. These are your feelings, they are legitimate and allowed. Experience them and let them go. You might need to repeat this process a few times.

Processing emotions is not usually a onetime event. Use your journal to pour out your emotion. Talk to a friend or therapist about any disturbing memories and feelings. Acknowledge that you have a right to your feelings. Accept your feelings as legitimate and natural. If you have intensely distressing emotions or flashbacks, please seek help from a therapist or an organisation such as The Samaritans or MIND.

If you are dealing with a more recent event or situation that has brought up anger for you, you could ask yourself questions such as:

- Why am I reacting to this situation/person/event with such intensity?

- What is my part in this situation?
- What action can I take to shift the anger–I could work it off physically, pour out my feelings into writing, write a letter or draft an email to someone to express anger (but not send it).
- Resolve to follow an appropriate plan of action, detach yourself from your angry feelings and when you feel calmer follow through on your plan.

By 'detaching from your anger' I am not suggesting that you deny it. I mean, look at it as if it is a separate entity to yourself. Imagine it as a rock or an object you are looking closely at, analysing, observing and noticing patterns. You are not your anger. Anger will come and it will go. Observe it with interest and compassion. Have compassion for yourself and if possible for anyone else involved in the situation.

To illustrate these points, I will give a personal example. Like many people in my teens and twenties, I felt a lot of anger towards my parents. The rage about various events and circumstances of my childhood was just below the surface most of the time.

I was generally considered a calm, even-tempered person – that was until someone ruffled my feathers and the anger would flare up rapidly with an alarming intensity. This was probably shocking for people closest to me.

Over time, I learned about observing my anger more objectively, feeling it but not allowing it to completely take over. I also learned to be compassionate towards myself and my parents. I saw that they genuinely did the best they could. Over time, the anger abated. I have found that if I ask myself questions about my reactions, I will usually find some interesting answers that are much more helpful than allowing myself to be subsumed by the emotion. I can't control other people's behaviour, but I can control how I respond to it.

It might be helpful to look back at the section in week three on 'Letting Go'. Remind yourself of the practical ways you can process difficult emotions and let them go. Remember, this will be a process and will take time. Be gentle and patient with yourself.

3. Fear

Fear exists to protect us. Without fear, we would injure ourselves or put ourselves into unnecessary danger. Healthy fear serves a purpose and keeps us safe. However, you may have grown up in a home where you were taught to be fearful of everything. Usually, this is not deliberate on the part of your caregivers. Over-protection and dire warnings about strangers, new situations, or taking any sorts of risks, are born out of love and care, not to be cruel or frightening. Unhealthy fear can stop us from making decisions and trying unfamiliar things. It feels safer to just stay at home and eat rather than go out into the big scary world and do new things. Binge eating can numb the fear. Like Maria, you might have been told as a child that the world is unsafe and dangerous. We can trust no one. Food is safe; we can rely on its comfort.

See fear for what it is, an instinct. Unhealthy fear is a fear that has got all bent out of shape. It needs to be downsized to realistic and manageable proportions. Fear need not run your life.

Look at the fear you feel today. Is the fear rational? Is it truly a life or death situation in the present moment? Probably not. Your fear is probably rooted in the messages you were given as a child about the world and how unsafe it is.

Consider fear in your life. What makes you afraid? Have you made decisions or choices that were driven by fear? Fear can appear to be something else; insecurity, anger, shame, or feelings of inadequacy.

When you are feeling fearful, how do you behave? Are you arrogant or humble? Do you feel you have to manipulate or control others to get your needs met?

For people with eating disorders or food issues, there may be specific fears such as:

- Fear of foods. Certain foods may make you feel very uncomfortable.
- Fear of not knowing who you are without the disordered patterns of eating.
- Fear of relinquishing such tight control over food.
- Fear of weight gain.
- Fear of losing a 'best friend' whether that 'friend' is food or an eating disorder.
- Fear of social events.

Take a moment to consider if you have any of these specific fears.

Note down in your journal the answers to these questions and reflect on their answers. Accept any feelings of fear you might have at the moment.

There is no need to rationalise or deny the fearful feelings. The answers to these questions will give you insights into how you have learned to be fearful, what triggers fear, how you deal with it and specific issues around eating. See these answers as useful insights into what might control your impulses and behaviour.

4. Shame

Shame has two sides. We can experience healthy guilt; the feeling we have when we know we have let ourselves down. This can spur us on to resolve to behave better next time. It can be the impetus to improve and move on. The other side is an unhealthy shame.

As a child, you may have been given the message from your caregivers, that you were not worthy of respect or love. You might have been told, either overtly or implied, that you were not wanted, that you were a burden. Perhaps there was abuse in the home or the family. You might have felt that somehow it was your fault and taken on this unhealthy shame. You believe that at heart you are terrible. You might experience agonizing self-doubt and feelings of inadequacy.

Self-compassion is an effective antidote to feelings of shame. In the introduction, I referred to the inner-critic. You remember that the inner critic is that voice that points out all your faults, shortcomings or mistakes. When you are assailed by the inner critic, replace it with the 'compassionate observer'. Imagine you are looking at yourself as you would look at someone you care deeply about and want to encourage and support them. You would not speak harshly to a cherished friend or a loved one if they were upset about a mistake or imperfection. You would try to be supportive and kind. Direct these same feelings towards yourself when you feel the inner critic attacks you.

You may experience intense shame because of trauma experienced as a child. If you have experienced the trauma of abuse as a child, please seek help. Working effectively through the effects of abuse is outside the parameters of this book but by being mindful of your feelings, you can start the journey towards health and healing.

If you have experienced trauma or painful experiences in the past, the words of the wonderful Gábor Máté might resonate with you:

''Unwittingly, we write the story of our future from narratives based on our past... Mindful awareness can bring into consciousness those hidden past based perspectives so that they no longer frame our worldview. Choice begins the moment you dis-identify from the mind and its conditioned patterns... In present awareness, we are liberated from the past.''(1).

In the meantime, use your journal to pour out your feelings about issues from your past you feel are affecting your present. Express all the pain of the child within you. Then resolve to be the adult who can take care of the child you were. You are the adult in control now.

5. Joy

Many people experience joy as a natural reaction to the delight they feel about their lives. This joy is genuine and comes easily. However, many other people use forced joy as a pretence to cover up emotions they feel they can't show the world. These are the people who run around after others, helping and smiling. No one can guess what is going on. When asked how they are, they will reply 'fine' with an enormous smile.

In your journal, write about all the things in your life, today, that truly gives you joy. If that is a struggle, write anything that comes to mind that has ever given you joy. Then write all the things you feel could give you joy. How often do you do these things? How many of them are centred on food or doing something for other people and expecting a return?

Permit yourself to feel all the range of emotions you will feel as a human being. Allow yourself to feel what you feel without trying to put on a smiling face for others. Open up to someone you trust and let them know how you are genuinely feeling. Most likely this person will be honoured to be trusted with your honest and open sharing. This helps build the intimacy and trust you have denied yourself.

This connection with others breaks the isolation and shame surrounding binge eating.

6. Emotional Check-ins

At points during the day, get into the habit of noticing your feelings. Try to name the emotion. Allow yourself to feel it without judging or blaming yourself. You need not talk yourself out of feeling the emotion or justify it. Just observe it and be aware of the effects that emotion has on your body and mind. For example, if you feel bored, you might notice that your energy levels feel low, you might feel inexplicably tired, you might move slowly and feel sluggish. Perhaps you feel the urge to sigh, your shoulders slump and you are yawning. Just notice and say 'I feel bored at the minute'. Accept that feelings will pass. Our feelings are just that–feelings. They are signals but not facts. We need not act on them right away. We need not try to change them with food or shopping or social media; we can just sit with the feelings and experience it rather than run away from it.

Try to see what the feeling is telling you about your life at the moment. Notice if the feeling has come as a reaction to a particular person, place, or thing. Bring a sense of curiosity to your noticing.

Establish this as a daily habit, regularly asking yourself 'How am I feeling right now?'

How to Deal with Difficult Emotions Mindfully.

1. Be aware of where you feel the emotion in your body. You might feel rage constricting your throat

or fear as a twisting sensation in your stomach. Accept the feeling, look at it and fully experience it.

2. Find a name for the emotion. Say to yourself; 'This is anger' or, 'This is fear.' Remember, you are not the anger or the fear, you are just feeling it.

3. Acknowledge the emotion and don't deny it

4. Remind yourself that feelings come and go. The feeling will pass, no matter how intense it feels.

5. Ask yourself some small questions about why this feeling has come up. If you don't know, just accept that you don't know. You might realise why you felt an emotion later. For example. I have had the experience of feeling unaccountably sad but at a later date realised that day was an anniversary of a loss.

6. Let go of trying to control your emotions. See them as interesting but transient, barometers of your experiences and reactions.

Note down any observations today in your journal.

I hope you have had time to listen to the guided meditation for this week. If not, take the time now to listen to the meditation for this week. Relax and enjoy it.

7. Summary

This week we have looked at the role emotions play in overeating or binge eating. We have established that everybody attaches emotions to eating at some time, or eats to feel comfort. However, with binge eaters, emotional eaters or chronic overeaters the difference is in the intensity, frequency and amount of food consumed. For binge eaters, overeaters or emotional eaters, eating enormous amounts of food becomes the only way to deal with emotions, not a once in a while indulgence.

We have gone into some detail looking at the key emotions that trigger overeating. It is important to feel and process these emotions, to break free from the cycle of overeating.

Being mindful of your emotions is a foundation of this work. Bring the attitudes of mindfulness to this awareness of your emotions. It might feel raw, to begin with, to experience feelings you have pushed down with food. But they are just feelings.

When experiencing your emotions, bring the attitudes of compassion and acceptance. Our emotions do not always make sense. Sometimes we can't rationalise them. Accept them just as they are. You need not justify them.

Approach your emotions with a sense of curiosity. Ask yourself 'what am I feeling?' regularly. Sometimes our emotions can surprise us.

Get into the habit of taking appropriate action to help soothe uncomfortable feelings such as shame or fear. Get support. Talk to friends and family and share your feelings. Mindfulness is about noticing the emotion. You don't have to stay stuck in a quagmire of uncomfortable feelings. Do what you need to do to feel more comfortable, this could mean moving in a way you enjoy, listening to music, picking up an absorbing craft or hobby, reading an uplifting book or planning a trip or event you are excited by.

By changing your behaviour in reaction to difficult emotions, you will form new habits that will have a powerful effect on your self-esteem and physical and emotional health.

If you feel you need to re-visit any of the sections this week, take the time to do so now. You have completed some challenging but necessary work this week. This takes courage and commitment. Take a moment to acknowledge the strength and determination you have shown this week.

Week Five

Self-esteem

When you believe in yourself more than you believe in food, you will stop using food as if it were your only chance at not falling apart. **Geneen Roth.**

Maria wondered why Sam stayed with her. He had such a sunny, easy-go-lucky personality. She felt intense and serious next to him, like a cold, damp shadow on a sunny day. When she shared these thoughts with him, he always brushed them away. She was being silly, and he loved her. Sam was tall and slim. She envied him. He could eat all he wanted and never put on a pound. Maria always seemed to be on a diet. She had been dieting since she was about twelve. The truth was Maria had always felt fat. Even her own mother had called her fat. Her mother had been a tiny person. Even as a teenager, Maria had felt like an elephant next to the little woman who linked arms with her daughter. Her heart sank, as Maria realised that for most of her life she had felt fat and ugly. No wonder she turned to cakes, chocolate, and sweets. They have given her the comfort she was desperate for.

Meditation for Self-Esteem

Let yourself settle comfortably on a mat or in a well-supported chair. Take a few deep breaths to relax and let go. Bring your attention to what you can sense around you. Be aware of the textures of clothing touching your skin.

Close your eyes and be aware of the colours behind your closed eyelids, Move your tongue around the inside of your mouth and focus on the taste in your mouth. As you breathe in, which aromas or scents do you detect?

Observe all of this with complete acceptance. If you have an aversion or resistance to how your experiences are at the moment, just notice it. Bring an attitude of acceptance to your circumstances today. Sit with this intention of complete acceptance.

Now bring this attitude of acceptance to yourself. Accept how you are in this moment, completely. You need not worry about changing or striving to improve. By gently moving forward one day at a time, moment by moment, making decisions that serve you well, you will grow and develop as you need to.

Accept that you are enough today. Say the words quietly to yourself: 'I am enough.'

Accept that you have enough today. Say the words quietly to yourself; 'I have enough'

Accept that this moment meets all your needs. Say the words quietly to yourself; 'This moment is enough'.

Bring to mind your qualities. This could be a skill, a personal attribute or ability. If you struggle with this, sit in silence and see what comes into your mind.

Imagine a scene in which you are with a dear friend, a loved one or a supportive and loving family member. Imagine how they might describe you. Imagine how they might feel when they are with you. In your mind's eye, see them smiling at you, expressing their warm feelings for you. Let feelings of appreciation and love for who you are, sweep over you.

Put your right hand over your heart and bring to mind attitudes of compassion, acceptance and gratitude for who you are.

Stay this way for a few moments.

When you are ready, stretch and move slowly, continuing with your day with a sense of self-love and acceptance.

1. B.I.N.G.E

The word 'binge' could be an acronym for (1):

Because

I'm

Not

Good

Enough

This could be: not pretty enough, clever enough, nice enough, smart enough, thin enough, fit enough and so on. Binge eaters often have a deep-rooted sense that somehow they lack the qualities and attributes that other people seem to take for granted. There is a deep sense of shame. We will discuss shame next week.

Where does this sense of not being enough come from? Why do people feel a sense of inadequacy about themselves they feel can only be comforted by food?

When a baby is born into the world, they do not see themselves as separate or distinct from other people. They are innocent of ego. To put it another way, they have no self-concept.

At around two years of age, that self-concept or ego forms. This is a delicate phase. Our idea of who we are is forming. If we are told we are loved, our mistakes or errors are seen as lessons in growth and learning and we are praised, we feel good about who we are. Sadly, many young children do not get these messages of support or encouragement from early caregivers. If our mistakes or errors are heavily criticised or if we are mocked, harshly scolded and punished unreasonably for minor indiscretions, we may grow up with the idea that who are is shameful and just not good enough.

Some people are more sensitive than others. Even reasonable chastisement or discipline could be perceived as damaging criticism by very sensitive children who do not have the life experience or self-regard to put such criticism into perspective. Often sensitive children grow up into sensitive adults. For some people, it feels as if there is never enough – enough food, enough love, enough attention, enough money, and enough happiness. Hoarding foods for a binge can give a false sense of comfort and reassurance, that, at least in the area of food, there is enough. However, as anyone knows who has tried this, enough is never enough. Cake and ice-cream can never satisfactorily fill this deep sense of shame and lack.

Messages around food could compound the effect of these early childhood experiences, for example, using sweet treats as rewards for good behaviour. As adults, we might reward ourselves with some forbidden food as a treat for a hard day at work. If we are feeling stressed or anxious, we might turn to the biscuit tin as a way of coping as we feel we do not have enough inner resources to cope in alternative ways. However, there is hope. We can learn that we are enough, just as we are right now. We can learn other ways of coping and self-soothing to deal with the challenges life throws our way.

I hope you have enjoyed the guided meditation today.

In your journal, please reflect on your past childhood experiences. By that, I mean your earliest memories up to about the age of seven or eight. Was food used as a reward? Did you feel supported and encouraged as a child or where you routinely scolded and shamed? Perhaps your memories fall somewhere in the middle? This is not about assigning blame on your past caregivers. People can only do what they can do. Look at their actions with compassion and acceptance, if you can. Try to look at your memories with a sense of objectivity and curiosity.

Just make a few notes of what strikes you about your memories. What messages were you given as a child about food, your body and diets? Do you feel your self-esteem was helped or harmed by your upbringing? Use your journal to unburden yourself of powerful emotions.

This exercise can bring up difficult emotions. Remind yourself that these are just thoughts and feelings. Sit with the feelings that come up. You may experience anger, resentment or grief. Look back at last week's section on emotions and use what is useful to you. Look again at week three; the sections on 'Letting Go' and 'Compassion'.

You are brave and courageous; a huge well done on completing this exercise today.

Tomorrow we look at how people-pleasing can affect self-esteem.

2. People Pleasing.

Compassion is central to mindfulness practice. I have encouraged you to practice compassion for others and yourself.

Today, we will look at how we balance compassion with our own needs. I am keen that you do not confuse compassion with people-pleasing.

By people-pleasing, I mean behaviour which puts our own needs last. It could be overt people-pleasing. Overt people-pleasing looks like this: people who are constantly running around after other people, turning themselves inside out to do what they think will make the other person happy. Alternatively, it could be covert people-pleasing, making important decisions based on what you think other people want.

There is nothing wrong with being agreeable or helping others. However, as a binge-eater whose self-esteem has been battered by feelings of shame and a lack of trust in your own judgement, it is easy to fall into the trap of constant people-pleasing.

People-pleasing can be about procrastination. You put other peoples' needs first to avoid doing what you know you need to do for yourself. This is a form of self-sabotage – you never get to practice a skill such as dancing or painting because you are just too busy looking after other people. You then lose sight of all the wonderful things you are capable of and your self-esteem becomes enmeshed in body image, diets and numbers on a scale.

Mindfulness practices, such as being aware of your feelings and tuning into your emotions, can help you identify your own needs. Your needs may have become subsumed by the desires of other people. You might feel unable to speak up for yourself. You might feel overwhelmed by rage or fear, which you keep stuffing down with food. You might try to stop the floodgates of emotion raging through your life by using food.

By being present to your feelings and learning to accept them, you can work out what is going on for you at a deep level. Use your mindfulness journal to write, without judgement or criticism. Then you can unpick the complex web that has got you all tangled up.

By paying attention to your reactions and emotions with curiosity, you can clarify what you need. By working this out and doing what you need to do to meet your needs, you see that the compulsion to fix yourself with an entire cake or box of chocolates will diminish.

By focusing on your feelings with a sense of self-compassion and acceptance, you are giving yourself the gift of respect for yourself. You may have behaved in the past in a way that seemed to say 'I don't care about myself.' You may have put yourself last at every opportunity. This has eaten away at your self-esteem slowly and sneakily. Now, it is time to identify and meet your needs, to give yourself the attention and dignity you have denied yourself for so long.

By practising self-compassion you will have no room for people-pleasing behaviour. If you are someone who never says no to extra work dumped on them at the last minute by their boss and who goes home to a family who expects you to do everything for them, you are not practising self-compassion. Reflect on what is going on for you at work, at home, and in relationships, right now. Do you say no, if you need to? Do you speak up and give your opinion, even if it differs from the other person? Do you let people know if you are too tired, too ill, or unable to complete a task, or do you just plough on, regardless? Observe your own behaviour and spot any people-pleasing that might be going on.

We can still practise compassion for others whilst balancing that with self-compassion. Being compassionate is not being a victim. We can have an attitude towards others that wishes them well.

By attending to your own needs, you can have more space to feel compassion for others. Your compassionate feelings for others won't be drowned out by weariness and a feeling of being a martyr. Your compassion will come from a deep and well-resourced reserve.

Sadly, people pleasers can irritate other people with their constant fussing and busyness. People feel uncomfortable around people pleasers. Often they don't respect people pleasers and ignore them or take them for granted. These responses make the binge eater feel even less worthy than they already did. People-pleasing backfires and has the opposite effect, they aren't pleasing anyone and are hurting themselves. This sense of being disliked or ignored can take the binge eater right back to a binge.

If compassion moves you to take action to help someone else, that is a wonderful thing. However, pay attention to your motives. Are you moved by genuine compassion or are you trying to be liked, accepted or wanted?

Be aware of people in your life who expect you to pick up after them, who regularly expect you to take on a task with short notice that will inconvenience you, who disregard your needs or wishes. Think about your responses. By always agreeing to do as they ask, you are not practising compassion; you are practising people-pleasing. Set boundaries with these people and expect them to do their share.

If it is time to set some boundaries, you may say no calmly and gently. Notice how you feel when you have to say no or when you disagree with someone. Breathe deeply, ground yourself and remind yourself that you have the right to practise self-compassion.

Spend some time thinking about the questions raised in this section today. Make a note of any people-pleasing you may be doing. And set some boundaries for yourself. This will take courage and it will feel difficult at first, but keep going. You will probably get some negative reaction, but stay steady. You are doing this to get well.

3. Self-Care/Resourcing

This week's focus is on building self-esteem. I would like to introduce self-care as an act of appreciation for yourself.

Perhaps you feel you need to be constantly doing things for other people, how can you take time out to pamper yourself?

Binge eating is an isolating experience. Perhaps your thoughts are orientated on yourself and you feel trapped in an endless cycle of self-loathing and harsh criticism of yourself. If this is the case you might look at practical things you are doing for yourself to help you feel better. Do you cook proper meals for yourself? Try focusing on cooking a nutritious and enjoyable meal, something simple like fixing a colourful salad or a sandwich made with delicious ingredients, set a place for yourself at the table, use your best crockery. Do this simple act for yourself as gratitude for your life and the ability to move and prepare a meal. Eat the meal with full attention on the taste, texture, and the look of the food.

I refer to 'resourcing' activities. By resourcing, I mean activities that make you feel better about yourself and your life. Essentially these are healthy activities, sustaining and nourishing to body, mind, and spirit.

By doing pleasant, resourcing things for ourselves we help establish a positive loop of trigger, behaviour, reward. For example, by preparing a nutritious meal you are making an effort to feel better by eating some healthy, enjoyable food; your positive emotions are the reward to repeat this more healthful behaviour.

Sometimes the act of self-care takes more discipline than we apply to our work life. Self-care is not all about massages and spas. Perhaps pushing yourself gently to go out for a walk or set aside ten minutes to organise your desk, are activities that will ultimately make you feel better.

Here are some ideas to get you started: Please note, if you do anything online, steer clear of anything associated with diets, diet culture, or extreme exercise.

- Go for a walk in nature.
- Phone a friend for a chat.
- Have a cup of your favourite hot beverage and savour it.
- Listen to uplifting music.
- Plan a day trip, a weekend away, or a holiday.
- Sort out your closet.
- Visit an art gallery.
- Buy yourself some flowers and enjoy arranging them.

- Pick up a hobby you used to enjoy–martial arts, painting, singing, dancing, etc.
- Write three things you admire about yourself or that you are grateful for.
- Go birdwatching.
- Take photos in nature.
- Create a vision board.
- Spend twenty-minutes watching an inspirational video.
- Try a new recipe.
- Colour, doodle or sketch.
- Lie down with a face mask on.
- Watch a comedy.
- Go for a swim.
- Sort out the photos on your computer.
- Make a greetings card–either using paper or digitally.
- Arrange a zoom call with a group of old friends from school, university, or a previous workplace.
- Look up and read inspiring quotations.

This is not selfish. By doing things for yourself that are sustaining, enriching, and healthful, you are building yourself up to be purposeful and useful to yourself and others.

Further ideas for self-care

Self-care can be divided up into eight categories; I present them as a list with suggested activities. Some of these will overlap, for example, going for a hike in the mountains would fall into the categories of physical well-being, awe-inspiring, practising a cognitive skill such as map reading and orienteering, solitude, or connection, depending on your needs and preferences.

Your self-care ideas will need to fit in with your likes, abilities, and personality. More introverted people will need more alone time than extroverts who need lots of opportunities to be with others. Try to attain a balance that works for you. Start small. Make consistent efforts and keep it simple.

Be intentional with your self-care activities. They won't happen by accident. The chances of you doing the activities are stronger if you have written them into your diary or onto your calendar. Try putting a reminder on your phone to prompt you to do a small act of self-care each day. By approaching self-care in this systematic and comprehensive manner, we can avoid much anxiety or feelings of overwhelm as life feels more balanced and manageable. You will then be less inclined to fall into the trap of feeling the need to binge eat or eat seeking a sense of comfort.

Physical well-being.

- Movement (walking, jogging, horse-riding, dancing, cycling, swimming).
- Sleep and rest–including naps and good sleep hygiene.
- Food and hydration.
- Alcohol limits.
- Limits on screen time.
- Massage.

- Haircut.
- Facial.
- Hot shave.

Creativity.

- Crafts.
- Art.
- Gardening.
- D.I.Y.
- Decorating.
- Flower arranging.
- Sewing.
- Photography.
- Card making.
- Baking a cake.
- Carpentry.
- Writing poems or stories.
- Writing a song or a piece of music.
- Creating a collage or vision board.

Cognitive/mental.

- Learning a language.
- Reading.
- Games.
- Quizzes.
- Teaching a skill.
- Learning a new skill.
- Skill swapping.
- Playing a sport that requires mental effort such as golf.

- Setting goals.
- Making plans.
- Learning to play an instrument.

Awe/Inspirational.

- Getting out into nature.
- Reading inspirational books.
- Spiritual pursuits such as attending church or praying.
- Spending time with animals.
- Listening to talks and podcasts that are uplifting.
- Watching nature documentaries.
- Looking at the stars and moon.
- Looking up at the sky every day.

Work/ Sharing skills.

- Meaningful work.
- Voluntary work.
- Sharing a skill.
- Babysitting for a friend or relative.
- Studying.
- Making instructional videos.
- Teaching a language.
- Setting work or career goals.
- Being a mentor or finding a mentor.
- Asking for feedback.

Connection.

- Ringing a friend or loved one.
- Writing a letter or card.
- Writing an email.
- Sending some photos.
- Hugging a loved one.
- Giving a small gift.
- Being present.
- Joining a club/church/group.
- Starting or taking part in a self-help group.

Emotional/mindfulness.

- Being present most of the time.
- Taking time out just to 'be'.
- Slowing down.
- Writing in a journal.
- Pausing to appreciate.
- Doing kind acts.
- Acknowledging emotions.
- Practising attitudes of mindfulness.
- Silence.
- Solitude/alone time.
- Hugging a loved one or a pet.

Organisational/time/money.

- Organizing a closet or drawer.
- Cleaning and tidying.
- Washing the car.

- Being aware of finances and spending.
- Avoid borrowing money.
- Budgeting.
- Setting financial goals.
- Writing realistic to-do lists.
- Keeping a diary/calendar.
- Arrange for some help if needed.

Pick out some activities that you would like to try. Enjoy!

4. Mindfulness for Self-Esteem

In Day 1 this week, we looked at how our childhood experiences can contribute towards feelings of not being enough ourselves or feeling that there is never enough of what we need.

By practising mindfulness, we can be more aware of these feelings. By being more aware, we have more of a chance of gaining some mastery over these feelings. We can experience them, look at them, and decide how we will process these feelings in a way that has the best outcomes for ourselves. We can make decisions that are in our best interest in terms of our mental and physical health.

Alternatively, if we operate from a basis of reacting automatically to our feelings with no awareness, we will follow the same conditioning. We have learned through influences around us and by reinforcing our behaviour, that if we feel inadequate, eating food for emotional comfort will, in the short term, take away these feelings. We carry on doing the same thing repeatedly, even though on a rational level we don't want to do it. By rushing headlong through each day and grabbing what we need to feel better temporarily, we just perpetuate the behaviour we want to stop.

Mindfulness teaches us to **Stop. Look and listen**.

When you feel tempted to binge, do just that: **Stop.**

Stop what you are doing. Just pause. You can eat the food if you really want to. No one is telling you what to do. But just take a moment. Now, look at yourself as if looking at another person. Imagine you are looking at someone you love and care about deeply. Is this behaviour that you would want for them? Look at what is going on at this moment. How are you feeling?

Look around at your immediate environment. Just notice what is going on. Listen to the surrounding sounds.

Listen to what is going on in your own heart and soul. What 'want' is the wanting of the food really about? What do you need right now at this moment? Do you need a hug, a chat with a friend, to sleep, to relax, a foot rub, a warm bath, a gentle walk, some quiet time, to feel uplifted or cheered up? What is it you genuinely need?

By practising mindfulness in this situation of being confronted by the urge to binge, you can get to the heart of what you truly need to feed, not just your belly but, your soul.

On a day-to-day basis, develop a habit of asking yourself at points: 'what do I need right now?' Ask yourself regularly: 'How am I feeling?' If you are hungry go right ahead and eat if that is genuinely what you need. Enjoy the food and be grateful for it.

Practice mindful eating as we talked about in Week 1, Day 6. Get to know what it feels like to be genuinely hungry. You need not wait until you are ravenous or feel light-headed because of low blood sugar, but make friends with the gentle sensation of a slightly rumbling stomach. Where I grew up, there is an expression: 'Hunger is the best sauce.' When we have moderate hunger, we enjoy simple food.

By taking these practical steps and feeling like you have some control over food, your self-esteem will grow. You will teach yourself alternative habits of responding to your emotions and needs in healthy ways. This will feed your self-esteem and give you confidence for the future.

Mindfulness can improve self-esteem.

In 2013, Christopher Pepping carried out research at Griffith University, Australia. He studied two groups of students. The group who were given fifteen minutes of mindfulness training each day showed higher self-esteem. The research group concluded:

"Mindfulness may be a useful way to address the underlying processes associated with low self-esteem, without temporarily bolstering positive views of oneself by focusing on achievement or other transient factors. In brief, mindfulness may assist individuals to experience a more secure form of self-esteem."

Rather than linking self-esteem to what we are good at or what we can do well, by practising mindfulness we are honouring ourselves in a much more sustainable way.

Mindfulness practices such as self-compassion can help build the self-esteem that gets eroded with the shame of food binges. What does self-compassion look like? Here are some ideas to get you started:

- Being kind to yourself; if you make a mistake, forgive yourself, learn from it, and move on.
- Be patient with any flaws you perceive in yourself.
- Be tolerant of any shortcomings you think you have.
- See your feelings within the context of being human–everyone feels inadequate sometimes and makes mistakes.
- Accept your feelings and don't tell yourself you 'shouldn't' feel something.
- Give yourself enough time to get things done.
- Don't expect perfection from yourself or anyone.
- Adopt a mantra of 'progress and not perfection'.
- Keep your responses to any shortcoming or failure within a moderate balance.
- Watch your inner self-talk. Is it kind?
- Attend to your physical and emotional needs promptly. If you are thirsty, drink water if you are hungry, eat a snack, if you are tired, take a break, if you need some company or a chat, talk to a friend or loved one. This seems basic but so many of us push on and on to complete projects or get a job

done, to the detriment of our physical and/or mental health.

- Be open to feedback and see criticism as a way to improve.
- When you see yourself in a mirror, pick out one or two things you like about your appearance.
- Eat top quality food. Don't damage your body with drugs, smoking, and excessive amounts of alcohol. Get enough sleep. Respect and nurture your physical self.
- Take time out to be in nature, meditate, stretch, and rest.

Today, think about how you practice self-compassion. In your journal, write some ideas that appeal to you and resolve to incorporate them into your life regularly. If this is hard for you, try just one slight change. This could be as simple as deciding to challenge your inner critic when self-criticism creeps in. For example, if you make a mistake or have a minor accident such as dropping a cup or plate, remind yourself that these things happen to everyone sometimes. Be kind to yourself.

I hope you have listened to the guided meditation on self-esteem today.

Remember to reflect on how far you have come. Give yourself credit for the work you are putting in to get well and stay well.

5. Acceptance and Control

Earlier in the book, we saw that acceptance is not a passive act of resignation but an active choice. We can decide to accept something.

Today, practice accepting yourself, just as you are. There might be aspects of your life that you want to change. See these urges as motivation to carry on with your efforts to get well and then let them go. These nudges to change can help you move on, grow and develop but they have served their purpose, now you need to drop the constant desire to be something different and accept yourself just as you are. Acceptance is part of moving forward. We are not fighting or striving; we are practising being content in our own skin, just for today. Life will change and move on. We can flow from one day to the next practising these mindfulness attitudes and behaviours and the changes will follow.

If you struggle with overeating, binging, or the perception of yourself as heavy and unattractive, all these issues will not be healed by fighting with them. By accepting the feelings or thoughts as just feelings or thoughts that have no power over you, you are in control. Don't let the thoughts dominate your day. They are just thoughts.

When you look in a mirror, accept your appearance just as it is. Be grateful for yourself as a unique human being. Don't let the inner critic take over. Replace the inner critic with the inner-nurturer.

Regularly tune in to how you are feeling internally. Do regular informal body scans to check in with the sense of who you are under the skin. Our appearance is just how we see ourselves in the mirror. It is only one aspect of all that makes you who you are. Keep it in proportion. Be mindful of all the sensations inside your body. Keep track of stress levels, hunger levels, and emotions. By checking in with yourself often, you avoid getting over-hungry. You can be aware of certain emotions building up and take appropriate action.

However, you are feeling, accept it. You may or may not like it, either way, just accept it for now.

By practising acceptance, we experience peace. These feelings of peace and contentment can fill the void we have used food to fill. If you do feel a fresh sense of peace, breathe into it and relish it.

In your journal make a note of anything you find difficult to accept about your body, appearance or situation at the moment. Without force, practice willingness to accept whatever issue it is for you. Be open to possibilities.

6. Practical Tips

In the last section, we looked at how practising mindfulness can help raise self-esteem, in particular, we looked in some detail at how practising compassion can help us feel better about ourselves at an intrinsic level that goes beyond being proud or pleased with ourselves for achievements.

Taking pleasure in our accomplishments is acceptable. I would encourage you to celebrate the achievements meaningful to you. However, the feeling can be transitory.

We want to encourage deep, unshakable self-esteem at the core of our being. By basing self-esteem on how well we do our job or how effective we are at parenting, a failure in these areas could have us spiralling down into a morass of self-doubt and questioning.

Other practical tips to build self-esteem are:

- Be you. Be your authentic self as much as you can.
- Move. Do whatever makes you feel good in your own skin–walk, jog, dance, stretch, garden, play with the kids, and play with your dog.
- Adopt a growth mind-set–you can learn from mistakes.
- Focus on what is within your control–more about this later.
- Celebrate all your successes no matter how small.
- Surround yourself with people who are supportive, kind and positive.
- Attend to your physical, mental and emotional health and avoid extremes.
- Be aware self-esteem is an 'inside job'. No one can give it to us. Invest in yourself and in all your efforts to build your self-esteem.
- Spread your interests and passions; don't just focus on your appearance. Learn new skills such as playing a musical instrument, learning a language, or drawing still-life.
- Adopt practices such as meditation, nature walks, quiet alone time, and journaling. These activities show self-respect. By taking time for yourself, you are learning ways to treat yourself kindly. How can

you have true self-esteem if you treat yourself more harshly than you would ever dream of treating another creature?

- Write yourself a letter of gratitude for all your personal qualities and attributes. Look at it when you feel low about yourself.

Use your journal to record one habit you will adopt to encourage a healthy, loving respect for yourself. This could be an idea listed above or something else that appeals to you. Above all, do it.

Show yourself some self-respect and compassion today by taking some time out to listen to the guided meditation. Spend a few minutes at the end of the meditation with a sense of gratitude and self-acceptance.

7. Summary

This week we have looked at the role self-esteem plays in overeating or binge eating. Often a vicious cycle is established: feelings of low self-worth can lead to overeating and the feelings of self-loathing can feed the low self-esteem. By interrupting this cycle with compassion and acceptance, you can break free from its miserable tyranny.

I hope you have found the practical tips useful to help repair your self-esteem. Go back now and have a look at them. Pick out a few to try. Perhaps, make a record of the tips you will put into action in your journal.

Which self-care activities have you tried this week? If you have found it difficult to find the time or motivation, try one thing within the next twenty-four hours.

To close today, I hope you are clear on the difference between practising compassion and the self-defeating people-pleasing that overeaters can get caught up in. Be mindful of your motivations and behaviour. Make any observation of note in your journal.

Hopefully, you have had time to listen to the guided meditations each day this week. If not, take some time now to listen to the meditation for this week. Relax and enjoy it. This is a gift of time and effort for yourself that will help you realise your self-worth.

Week Six

Body Image

There is something wonderfully bold and liberating about saying yes to our entire imperfect and messy life. **Tara Brach**

Maria slunk behind the others in the back row of the yoga class. The room was surrounded in mirrors. She saw herself as the round blob in black. All the other women and men attending the class were lithe and slim. Why was she even here? Maria suddenly felt desperate to leave. The yoga teacher was welcoming. Maria didn't want to appear rude. She struggled on for a few more minutes, and then suddenly stood up, gesturing to the pretend watch on her wrist and shaking her head apologetically. 'Sorry' she mouthed. Maria rolled up her mat and almost ran out of the door, smiling idiotically and waving, not wanting to offend the teacher. As she left the room her gaze settled on the vending machine. Some chocolate was just what she needed to settle herself. She scrabbled around for coins and pushed them into the machine urgently. Maria felt humiliated by the memory of how she looked in the yoga studio mirror. Her face felt feverish from shame.

Meditation on Appreciation for Your Body.

Allow yourself to relax back in the chair or on the mat. Make yourself as comfortable as possible and allow yourself to enjoy this time to relax. Approach the meditation with a spirit of curiosity. Be curious about what might come up for you today. Bring the attention to the breath. Observe the breath. Don't adjust, just watch it come and go. Now bring the attention to the feet. How are your feet feeling today? Reflect on all the ways your feet serve you. Think of all the distance your feet have walked or ran.

Focus now on your legs and hips. Consider how your legs and hips have moved to carry you around every day. Take a moment to be grateful for your feet and legs. Bring your awareness to the torso. Consider all the organs your torso houses. Reflect on how these organs function day after day to keep you alive and well. Be thankful for your vital organs that keep you in good health. Breathe fully into the belly and be thankful for any roundness or fullness in the belly. This shows it is full of life-giving air. Remind yourself that the belly is meant to be round and soft.

Be conscious now of your arms. Think of all the ways you use your arms- to reach, to pull, to push and to embrace loved ones. Think about your hands; bring to mind all the jobs your hands do day after day. Now focus on your face . and how you use your face to express emotion, to smile and laugh. Be thankful for the unique arrangement of features that is your face.

Be aware of the sensation of your head resting against the surface, supporting it. Be grateful for the protection your skull provides to the brain. Spend a few moments in awe at how complex and amazing the brain is. In this moment of appreciation for the body and mind, commit to nourishing your body and mind in the best ways possible, every day. If any resistance or aversion comes up, look at it dispassionately and let it go. Cultivate the idea that your body is your home – a home to be cared for and maintained like any physical home. Take a full breath and stretch, relish in the way your body feels as you stretch fully. Put your right hand over your heart and take a moment to thank your body for all that it does. As you carry on with your day, show an appreciation of your body by being mindful of its needs, attending to those needs and taking actions healthy to the body and mind. Move slowly and carry on with your day.

1. Perceptions and Perspective

Our perceptions as human beings can be very unreliable. Our perception can change from day to day. What seems perfectly fine one day can seem negative on another day. You can look in the mirror on any day and see an acceptable image or an unacceptable image. You might hear the inner critic and criticise your appearance harshly. Other people might see your lovely hair, beautiful eyes, or a pretty smile. Ultimately though, you are not the hair or the eyes or the smile. You are a person with feelings, desires, talents, qualities, and needs. Our bodies are fantastic vehicles that take us through life. They allow us to hug, dance, run and stretch. Yet we look on the outside of our bodies with judgement warped by our own unreliable and changeable perceptions and by the various images we are exposed to each day.

There is also a kind of cultural unreliability around perceptions of the body and physical appearance. What is seen as attractive changes over time. I am sure you can think of many examples of this. Some years ago, a comedienne got lots of laughs with her constant, worried question of 'Does my bum look big in this?' Nowadays it seems the bigger the better. Apparently, there is bottom implants surgery available. It just shows how crazy it all is.

Happiness with our bodies is an inside job. By feeling good in your own skin, happiness will follow. By treating our bodies and emotional selves with respect, compassion, acceptance, and gratitude we will drop the obsessive chase of striving for the perfect body to be happy. You cannot punish yourself into feeling good about your body.

Think about how unreasonable it is to judge ourselves against images of bodies that are not real. You might look in the mirror on an average morning and judge the image harshly, mentally comparing it to what you see in a magazine or on social media. These images are created by make-up artists, lighting technicians, and talented camera people. Then the image is most likely airbrushed and manipulated to give the desired result. It is not real. You are comparing yourself with an illusion. Be mindful of that.

When you look in the mirror find three things you are grateful for and that you like about your appearance. Do it often. When a critical thought enters your mind, dismiss it as 'Just a thought.' Smile at yourself in the mirror and appreciate how your eyes light up. Take a breath to feel a sense of gratitude and appreciation for your body.

Gratitude is a powerful mindfulness tool to overcome feelings of shame, repulsion, or criticism; practise being grateful for your body often. Treat it with respect and care. Take breaks when you need to, rest, give yourself good quality food, use the best products you can afford, move when you need to and practise self-care.

Treat your body with compassion. Don't wear uncomfortable shoes or restrictive clothing. Eat when you are hungry. Visit the dentist regularly and go for medical check-ups. Enjoy regular baths and showers using excellent quality products. Consider going for a massage or spa treatment. This isn't indulgent; it's taking responsibility for looking after yourself. Pay attention to what your body is telling you and take action to feel more comfortable. By investing in taking care of your body and respecting it, you are less likely to give in to the urge to treat it unkindly by cramming in masses of excess food that will ultimately harm your mind, body, and soul.

Wear clothes that fit you well and that are comfortable. Pay attention to the colours that make you feel bright and optimistic and chose textures that you enjoy the feel of. Don't wear clothes that are torn or stained, not even just around the house.

Make a note in your journal of aspects of your body you are grateful for.

2. Movement versus Exercise

For many people, exercise has become another way to punish the body. A binge eater might play some mind games with numbers, calculating the massive amount of effort needed to offset the calorific disaster of a binge. A long run or cycle ride is planned to burn off calories and not for the joy of being able to move one's body and enjoy the endorphins.

Gruelling gym sessions might be followed by a 'justified' huge takeaway and/or chocolate hit. This attitude towards movement is another side effect of the diet culture. How often have you started a diet with an intensive exercise regime only to give up on both due to hunger and exhaustion?

Movement can make us feel good, improve our mental acuity, build and maintain muscle mass, maintain bone density and is great for the circulation.

 Don't wait until you are a certain size or weight to get involved in exercise. For exercise to be sustainable it needs to be:

1. Enjoyable – ignore statements like: 'No pain, no gain.'
2. Simple – complicated regimes are not sustainable.
3. Time-efficient - most of us do not have time for a two-hour gym session.
4. Cheap or free – there are lots of free resources on YouTube. Dancing in your living room, walking, swimming in the sea or a lake, doing yoga or callisthenics at home are all free. In Appendix 2 of this book, there are some simple mindful movements to try.

Think about what is healthy and resourcing for you. Above all do what you enjoy.

Functional Movement

My grandmother, who grew up in a rural area in Ireland, used to tell me stories of how she had to walk five miles to school and five miles back. As a child, I walked at least two miles to school and two miles back. We had no car.

Nowadays, in most places, it would seem that most children get transported to school in cars. We go to the supermarket in a car, do errands in the car and drive to areas of natural beauty to sit in the car and eat chips or ice cream.

It would seem strange to my grandmother, to see people today, get in their cars to drive to a gym to walk or run on a treadmill, and pay for the privilege to do it. It would seem that our relationship with exercise has got as skewed as our relationship with food.

We were designed to move, to walk, to run, to stretch, to twist, to push, to pull, to lift, and so on. We need to move. However, we need not look on it as another chore, another item to tick off on a 'to do' list, or as something to assuage our guilt when we have overindulged. Instead of feeling you 'have to' exercise, find something you enjoy doing and do it. Don't link it to food. Don't do it to force your body into looking a certain way or to fit into clothing that has a certain size on it. Do it and just see what happens. Let go of the outcomes. Find something that puts you into the zone in which time flies by and you feel sad about finishing.

On a day-to-day basis, look for situations where it would be safe and convenient to walk. Build in a walk to go to the shops or do errands. Shop more locally and more frequently. You will support local businesses, getting to know people in your local area, and eating more sustainably. You will also use your time more productively.

You can practise mindfulness techniques as you walk to the shops. Look around your neighbourhood, listen to the sounds of the birds, get some fresh air, and move.

Instead of driving in your car, dashing around the supermarket and coming home to binge, take your time. Enjoy the stroll to the shops, speak with your neighbours, and feel a sense of connection with others and with your environment.

Think about how you can incorporate this into your life. Start small. Go a short distance, buy just a few items, and see how it feels.

Think about how you could incorporate some walking into your life. Dan Buettner studies populations around the world and identified what he has called 'blue zones', those are areas in the world where people live long healthy lives.

In Sardinia, a blue zone identified by Buettner, it is not unusual for people to live to be one hundred and still be active and independent. People in Sardinia don't 'exercise' – they move. They walk to get their groceries and carry them back. They grow produce and flowers and tend to their gardens. They clean their houses and bustle about the kitchen. They stroll out and chat with friends and

188

neighbours. No one rushes about, they enjoy the little things, they eat well, eating traditional, local foods' and they naturally build-in functional movement into their daily lives.

Consider how, where and when you could build in enjoyable, functional movement into your daily routine.

3. The Body-Mind Connection

Activities such as yoga or Tai Chi are good examples of how we can incorporate movement with mindfulness in a structured way. In the appendix, there are some suggestions for gentle movements based on yoga poses. These sorts of movements calm the mind, focus the attention, help with body awareness, and can help with a range of ailments or disorders.

Deep yoga stretches can help shift built-up tension in areas such as the hips and shoulders. Often this can provide emotional release. I have taught yoga for twenty years and have seen how its practice can bring on tearful emotional releases. As we have seen, intense emotional states, or trying to avoid them, can bring on a binge; a practice such as yoga is a healthier alternative in seeking this emotional release. Going to your yoga mat to gently stretch and move the body in a way that honours our physical self is much more nurturing and restorative than a gym session you have hated every moment of.

When practising yoga you become more mindful of moving with ease and grace. Why would you want to overstuff yourself with food and feel bloated and uncomfortable on the yoga mat and in your life? This is a matter of feeling comfortable and at ease.

There is no judgment or blame, just pleasure at feeling at home in our amazing body. Anyone can practise a gentle regimen of yoga, Tai Chi, or Chu Gong, no matter what size or fitness level. This is not about outcomes but about feeling more in tune with ourselves. It's about having respect and compassion for ourselves. If you feel the urge to binge, try going to your yoga mat instead, breathe, and move, release the emotions you are looking to let go of. If you can do this, your body, mind, and future self will thank you for it.

When practising mindful movement, whether a formal yoga or tai chi practice or gentle stretches, bring an attitude of gratitude. This could be a sense of gratitude for your body and its ability to move and stretch, gratitude for the time to practise or for an aspect of your surroundings.

Today, make a note in your journal of some small, simple ways you could build in movement into your daily routine. Make a note of any forms of movement or sports you've always wanted to try.

4. More on the Body Scan

So many of us rush through the day with little awareness of what is going on below our necks. We are so focused on mental lists and chatter: "Remember to pick up the dry cleaning, oh and while I head there I can stop off to pick up some groceries...what can I make for tea tonight? " And the endless chatter goes on. It's only when some part of our body begins to hurt that we might notice anything.

So many aches and pains come from extended periods of holding muscles tight with no respite that we begin to feel achy, tired and stiff. When we take a few moments to notice how we are feeling there is space for some re-adjustment, some relaxation and the avoidance of issues such as tension headaches, an aching jaw, shoulders that are so tight they are hunched up to your ears, digestive problems and aching joints.

The more that you practise body scans or body awareness the easier it gets. With time and practice, you will be able to do a body scan when you are travelling on public transport, in a long queue, waiting in the doctors or dentists. Play about with this internal awareness and attention on your physical sensations. You might start to notice patterns of how you hold yourself or move that explain that backache or neck stiffness.

It is easier to prevent tension from building up in the first place. The tricky bit is remembering to stop and take a moment to be aware of how we are feeling. The body scan helps with building this awareness that hopefully will become habitual.

By practising a body scan you can also feel like you have some control over your feelings. By stopping at points during the day and considering how you feel in your body, you can detect more subtle changes in how you are feeling. This allows you to take some action to avoid a build-up that can lead to a relief-seeking binge on food. For example, you might have a long drive home from work. Perhaps you usually get home, stiff and stressed from the drive and immediately dive into a tub of ice cream or put the kettle on and eat a packet of biscuits with your cup of tea. By being more mindful of your physical sensations you can take more healthful and beneficial measures such as spending five minutes stretching when you arrive home or running yourself a warm bath. Even lying down on the floor or a firm bed can help ease out the kinks in your back, neck and shoulders. Perhaps, your new routine could be to listen to a guided meditation for a few moments to help de-stress and relax after a long day.

Practise the body scan to get in tune with your natural hunger. You might have cravings for certain types of food but with practice and awareness of the signals your body is sending you, you will be able to tell the difference. When you are truly hungry you will have a sense of emptiness in the stomach and intestines, your stomach might make soft growling noises and you will have a rumbling sensation in your tummy. These are signs that you need to eat. If you are hungry, go ahead and eat. If you are not hungry you can wait for an hour and tune into your body and see if you are hungry yet. Don't wait until you are ravenous to eat. This may lead to overeating and feeling uncomfortably full.

5. Creating a Supportive Environment

Today, be mindful of what you have in your home that hurts your self-image or your chances of changing your behaviour in a more healthful direction.

In Week 1, I encouraged you to look mindfully at your environment and have a clear out. You may not have done this yet, so today or sometime this week is a good time to do it as you move forward with this mindfulness program. Look back at that section under the 'Practical Tips' heading.

By clearing out clothes that no longer fit, you are accepting the size you are today. Don't keep 'fat' clothes or 'thin' clothes that remind you of what you once were or what you might become. Keep your focus on the here and now.

By clearing out diet books and diet foods, you are freeing yourself up from the shackles of the diet industry and all its promises. You are now focussed on your behaviour, your emotions, and feelings, not on a number on a scale.

Clear off any diet-related apps on your phone. Unfollow any influencer or personality who is touting diets or extreme exercise programs.

Having an environment supportive of your mental and emotional health will help you feel better, be happier, and at peace.

Make your home calm and peaceful. Avoid having the television on around the clock. Play gentle music, keep your space as tidy and clutter-free as possible to help you feel relaxed and at ease. I understand that this is easier said than done if you have children at home or a busy family life. However, try to keep at least one room in the house as a place you can retreat to enjoy some quiet time.

6. Practical Tips

Today I will list some practical tips to consider which might help with body image:

- Change your focus from losing weight to changing your behaviour habits. By this I mean stop weighing yourself constantly and worrying about the numbers on the scale. Adopt behaviours such as eating well – that means eating enough and not skipping meals, moving regularly, sleeping well, and treating yourself with compassion and gratitude.
- Explicitly show your body gratitude by treating it well.
- Stop comparing yourself to others.
- Stop criticising yourself and pay no attention to the inner critic. See these as just thoughts.
- Use the guided meditations to help you feel positive and accepting of your body.
- Take opportunities to pamper your body. Use excellent quality products and take the time to attend to yourself.
- Clear out your wardrobe. No 'fat clothes', 'thin clothes', torn, stained, or uncomfortable clothes.
- Be mindful of your posture. Stand up straight. Walk slowly and as gracefully as you can.
- Know that any negative thoughts or feelings you might have about your body on any day should be seen in perspective. This can change from day to day.

- Be mindful of the material you are reading or looking at. Ask yourself if it supports your efforts to feel positive about your body and your life. If the answer is 'no' let it go.

Using your journal

Journaling can be a powerful tool in helping you develop patterns of thinking and reacting about your body and food. You can use your journal to write freely without any particular structure. If this feels difficult or you are not sure where to start, you can consider the following prompts:

- I feel most comfortable in my body when…
- When I think about my body the first thought that comes into my mind is…
- My body needs …
- When I think about my body I am grateful for…
- I find it hard to accept the following things about my body…
- The following things make my body feel good…
- My earliest memory of my body was when…

Lastly, I have a little acronym for you to recall when you look in the mirror: SMILE.

- Smile at yourself and others. It makes everyone feel better.
- Miracle – remind yourself often that your life is precious and miraculous.
- I am enough – you are complete and acceptable just as you are.

- Love -show yourself and others love and compassion.
- Enjoy – enjoy your body, stretch it, soothe it with warm baths and lotions, cocoon it in cosy clothing and use it to express love for others.

7. Summary

I hope that the practical tips will help you. They are a round-up of some behaviours and practices to build into your daily life.

It is also my hope that you will treat your body with compassion, care and kindness. Treat your body as your best friend. Nurture it and give it what it needs.

Consistency is key, keep doing them and they will become part of who you are. Make a note in your journal of any of the practices that appeal to you. Commit yourself to try out a couple.

Spend some time today considering your attitude towards your body; make a note in your journal of anything that comes up for you.

Remember to listen to the guided meditation today.

Take a moment to congratulate yourself on coming this far.

Week Seven

Stress, Anxiety and Depression

Don't believe everything you think. Thoughts are just that—thoughts. **Allan Lokos.**

Sunday evening always seemed to roll around too quickly for Maria. Her heart sank as she contemplated another week. She dreaded the daily grind of a 6.30 am wake-up, followed by the struggle to get the boys out of bed, rushing to get everyone in the car in time for school and work. She didn't even want to think about work. The house was quiet at the moment. The television was on in the living room and the kitchen was empty. Maria strolled in, wiped down the countertops, and opened the fridge. Just a few bites of something sweet would take the edge off her low mood. Maria rummaged around and found some chocolate mousse dessert. Just one, she thought, after all, I didn't have dessert today. She closed the kitchen door and sat down at the table to enjoy a few moments to herself. The first few bites of the desert seemed to ease her feelings of anxiety about the week to come. As she spooned it in more rapidly, her focus was not on the taste but on the mental pictures in her mind of what was coming up over the next week. She scraped away the last traces of the mousse in the pot and spooned it into her mouth, already on her feet, walking back towards the fridge...

Meditation for Relaxation

Only do this meditation when you can have a few moments to give it your full attention and can be undisturbed. Do not listen to this audio recording when operating machinery or driving.

Now, take a few moments to settle back into a comfortable chair or on a bed.

I will take you on a guided meditation to help you relax and let go. If you need to respond to any urgent situation, you will be able to do so. Please keep your focus on my voice, your breath, and the sensations in your body. If other thoughts come to mind, bring your focus back to my voice and the breath, and just let the thoughts go.

Ensure that you are warm and that your head is supported by a cushion or pillow. Make any adjustments you need to feel at ease and relaxed for about ten minutes. In a few moments, I will make suggestions to you to imagine a scene in your mind's eye. Don't worry if you don't immediately see a picture of what I suggest. Just have a sense of being in the place I suggest, using the sense or senses that work best for you.

For now, just breathe in deeply and slowly through the nose. You need not force the breath; just breathe slowly and deeply, breathing right the way down into the belly. Be conscious of the chest rising and the abdomen inflating.

Let the breath slowly release, be aware of the sensation around the nostrils. Deepening and lengthening the breath. Have a sense of ease and comfort. Allowing yourself this time for deep relaxation. The more you practice this deep relaxation, the more you will be able to handle the trials of life. You will feel more of a sense of control over the external and internal triggers and over the ebb and flow of emotions as you move through each day. You will be able to respond to these difficulties from a grounded centre of calm and equanimity.

Take a few moments to snuggle into the comfortable, safe place where you are now and enjoy a sense of peace and relaxation. If you are comfortable doing so, allow your eyelids to close softly.

Now bring your attention to the body, be aware of the points of contact your body makes with the chair or bed. Have a sense of the weight of your body, let your body feel heavy, loose, and limp as you relax back. If you are aware of any areas of tension, direct the breath to that area. As you breathe out, let the tension go.

Continue to breathe in deeply and as you breathe out, allow yourself to sigh gently and release any tension, negativity, discontent, anger, or upset. Gently letting it go.

Know that letting go is a process. Stay anchored in the breath, keeping the thoughts and awareness on a sense of relaxation, just allowing yourself to relax and be at ease in this safe space.

Remind yourself that at this moment all is well. You are safe, warm, and relaxed. There is no need to do anything or go anywhere right now.

In your mind's eye, imagine you are out in nature, in a grassy clearing at the edge of a wooded area. You can hear the wind rustling through the leaves on the trees and in the distance; you hear water trickling over rocks. You can feel the warm sun on your face and you have a sense of relaxation and warmth. You are barefoot and you can feel the soft grass beneath your feet. A body of water is glistening and twinkling in the sunlight. As you walk towards the water you can see and hear the water tumbling down over the rocks, forming a gushing waterfall into a peaceful lagoon.

You look forward to immersing yourself in the cool flowing waterfall. In your mind's eye, you move down towards the lagoon anticipating the cool crisp sensation on your warm skin. At the water's edge, you undress quickly and step into the lagoon. You are grateful for its cleansing and cooling effect. You immerse yourself, enjoying the refreshing sensation. You move through the shallow water, keen to get to the waterfall. You feel yourself glide along towards the waterfall. The sun glints off the cascading water, creating mini rainbows and sparkles as the crystal clear waterfall gushes down into the lagoon.

You make your way to stand under the falling water, enjoying it, massaging your head, neck and back. You have a sense of the water washing away any tension or emotional disturbance. You sigh as you enjoy the refreshing sensation on your skin. As you stand under the waterfall, your gaze settles onto the still surface of the lagoon. Its smooth surface reflects the glistening sunshine. You are mesmerised by the glassy stillness of the lagoon.

You are aware of the intense greenness of grass in the clearing by the edge of the lagoon. You have a contented sensation of peace and calm. Everything is just as it needs to be.

You make your way back through the water to the edge of the lagoon. You step out onto the grassy bank. There is a towel there that has been warmed by the sun. You dry yourself and relax back in the sunshine, sighing out deeply, enjoying these few moments of deep relaxation and calm. Focus now on this sense of relaxation and looseness, feeling heavy and warm, just letting every muscle in your body let go. Breathe into this sensation and remind yourself that this feeling of relaxation is available to you whenever you need it. If at any time you need to compose yourself, close your eyes for a few seconds and recapture this sensation of letting go and of deep relaxation. It is within your control to let go of any disturbing emotions or sensations at any time by using the power of your imagination. Reflect on this for a few moments and relish the calm comfort that you are experiencing.

Now, begin to focus again on the points of contact your body is making with the chair or bed at this moment. Deepen the breath and bring your awareness back to the here and now. Wiggle your toes and fingers and move your head gently from side to side. Take a breath in, perhaps raising the arms and giving yourself a refreshing full-body stretch.

Open your eyes, smile, and stand up slowly. Take this feeling of peace and contentment with you as you move through your day.

1. Mindfulness for Stress, Anxiety, and Depression

If you feel stressed or anxious, you may be interested in reading my book *Mindfulness for Stress and Anxiety.*

Stress has been named as the number one world health epidemic by the World Health Organisation. Today more people than ever report feeling stressed.

The stress response is a physiological reaction that has developed over millennia. We feel a threat and a serious of hormonal, chemical, and physical reactions take place to help us deal with that threat. However, the problem is the reactions often don't feel very helpful. Racing heart, a dry mouth, and an urge to run away or fight can feel disconcerting. Stress can be acute or chronic. Perhaps the stress response kicks in when we have a difficult commute to work once in a while, that's acute. If we live with an abusive partner and feel a constant sense of fear and anxiety, that is chronic stress.

Often, binge eaters will try to soothe the stress response with food. Denying emotions and carrying on, regardless. By bringing mindfulness practice to our day to day lives, we can see when and where we feel stress and anxiety and take constructive action.

In your journal, note down any situations in which you feel stressed or anxious. You might also want to review the notes you made in your journal in Week 5, Day 3 when we looked at fear.

2. BED and Stress, Anxiety and Depression

Stress affects everyone to a greater or lesser extent. Most people feel anxious at some stage in their lives, or have situations or events that provoke feelings of anxiety. Anyone can experience feelings of low mood or depression. However, binge eaters or people who have issues with overeating often have extra factors that bring on stress, anxiety or depression. 85% of binge eaters struggle with a mood or anxiety disorder.

Often binge eaters have grown up experiencing high levels of stress. A certain level of 'normal' stress is healthy for children. The stress of starting school or a change of teacher is part of growing up. Children need to build resilience and character. The key thing is that children need a consistent caregiver or nurturing adult to help support them with stress. If children experience extreme toxic stress such as war, abuse or parental substance abuse, without a reliable caregiver to support them, their stress levels will be constantly high. This constant surge of stress hormones means the child's brain develops differently. This will cause impulsivity and a desire for heightened experiences such as sugar rushes and risky behaviour.

Many binge eaters will have trauma in their backgrounds. This need to feel intense experiences can lead to a pattern of being attracted to extreme diets or patterns of eating and intense workouts. The brain development of people with childhood trauma means that dopamine levels are low. The excitement of a novel diet is intoxicating. The promise of reward in the form of thinness or a six-pack is enticing. The new program of obsessive calorie or point counting, special foods, food rules, measuring, weighing, restricting will be embraced with the anticipation of dramatic and rapid results. When this doesn't happen the resulting disappointment can lead to binge eating. In the introduction, I made the point that consistency trumps intensity. A slow, steady, sustainable approach is not as exciting, but it works in the long term. I hope that these observations help you understand why diets are so alluring and why they are such a major disappointment.

Environmental and social factors might heighten feelings of stress for binge eaters. People who have problems with eating may feel extra sensitive to societal pressures to be thin or to look a certain way. They can often be perfectionists who struggle to accept themselves as they are. Feelings of shame about the amount or type of food eaten can bring on feelings of anxiety, stress or depression.

In a study in Australia looking at what starts a binge, 91% of participants in the study reported tension as being the primary catalyst for a binge. (1). Therefore, it is essential people struggling with binge eating find ways to relax, self-soothe and care for themselves when feeling tense or stressed.

As noted yesterday, overeaters or binge eaters will turn to food as a comfort to deal with feelings of stress, anxiety or depression. The comfort food releases dopamine, which can help the person feel better for a short time. A habit of overeating highly palatable foods is then reinforced. What you will be doing is using mindfulness practices and other interventions to break this reward loop. You will find other ways to find comfort when you feel stressed, anxious or depressed.

This week we will look at a variety of lifestyle factors that could contribute to feelings of low mood, anxiety or stress. There will be lots of practical tips to help you relax, improve sleep quality and cope with stress and negative feelings.

By incorporating mindfulness practices into your life, you are helping to break the stress response as discussed yesterday. Tomorrow we will look at how stress chemical affects binge eating specifically.

I hope that yesterday you could make a note of any stresses in your life at the moment. If you didn't have time, take a few moments to do that now.

If you are suffering from debilitating stress, intense anxiety or chronic depression, please seek help from a qualified professional. You do not have to suffer alone.

Remember to listen to the guided meditation. Focus on making yourself comfortable and enjoy it. Use lots of cushions, blankets and perhaps an eye mask or eye pillow to feel relaxed. Enjoy the feelings of relaxation and comfort.

3. Stress Chemicals and Eating

Binge eaters have established a pattern of using food to deal with negative emotions. It is easy to get into a loop of feeling stressed and harassed, being too tired to practise meaningful self-care and turn to food as a quick 'pick-me-up'. Tomorrow we will look in more detail at the importance of adequate sleep quality to help with binge eating. Today we will look at some chemical reactions that happen when we are stressed or over-tired.

Stress releases high levels of cortisol. This in turns affects the levels of another hormone called ghrelin. Ghrelin is the hormone that tells us we are hungry. So the more stressed we feel, the hungrier we will feel. Cortisol also lowers another hormone called leptin. Leptin signals to our body feelings of satiety or fullness. Therefore, you might feel that your cravings are more intense when you feel tired or stressed.

Practising techniques such as meditation, mindful walking in nature, breathing with focus and attention and mindful eating, all help to lower the heart-rate and the release of stress hormones such as cortisol. This in turns affects the hunger/satiety hormones and consequently, cravings are reduced.

Taking time out for body scans is essential in dealing with stress or other negative emotions. You can then focus on what you need to do to feel more comfortable or calmer. Earlier, I talked about doing body scans to help identify genuine hunger. The practice is also important to identify thirst. Sometimes we mistake thirst for hunger. So having a drink of water is always a helpful first step if you feel unexpectedly hungry. Dehydration can also lead to the release of a hormone called vasopressin, which increases feelings of anxiety and depression. So having a drink of water can also help with these disturbing emotions. Be mindful of feelings of thirst and ensure you drink enough water, herbal tea or other non-caffeinated drinks.

Compassion and Connection.

We have looked at the importance of compassion towards ourselves and other people. This is an attitude we bring to daily life as we practice mindfulness. Connecting with others releases a hormone called oxytocin, sometimes referred to as the 'hug drug'. This hormone can help us feel happier and more connected with others. Oxytocin promotes a reduction in anxiety and depression. This underlines the importance of listening with full attention to others. By doing this we are showing our interest and concern for others which helps build the connections which release oxytocin. Even just smiling and greeting a stranger or patting a friendly dog can help release these feel-good hormones. We strengthen bonds with others and build our sense of self-esteem. These factors work together to help us feel happier and food becomes less of an issue.

I hope that this underlines to you the importance of self-care and soothing mindfulness practices. These are not just fluffy self-indulgences; they are part of a holistic package that can treat problem eating.

Take time today to be mindful of how you are feeling, especially in terms of thirst, fatigue and hunger. Take a few moments to reflect on your methods of relaxation. Are they resourcing? Reflect on your quality of sleep and your bedtime and morning routines. We will look at the link between sleep quality and binge eating in more detail tomorrow.

I am also giving you a gentle reminder to remember to listen to the guided meditation. Now that you are aware of the physiological effects of stress, anxiety and low mood on your eating habits, I hope you will prioritise relaxation and self-care as part of your plan to overcome binge eating or overeating.

4. Sleep Quality and Eating

There is a clear correlation between sleep issues and binge eating. Many people with disordered eating habits report problems with insomnia. As we noted yesterday fatigue can raise ghrelin levels and lower leptin levels, meaning we are more inclined to feel hungry and less satisfied with our food.

When we feel tired, we will often reach for higher-calorie foods, particularly sweet foods to help lift feelings of exhaustion. Cravings for high sugar, high-fat foods are intensified.

Can you relate to the following scenario?

Maria threw the bag of shopping onto the table and sat down heavily on the kitchen chair. Her feet hurt, and she felt like a hand was pressing down on her head. The sleepless nights and busy days at work and then chores at home were taking their toll. The thoughts of stirring herself to put away the shopping and prepare dinner were overwhelming. After a few moments, she sighed and stood up wearily. Sam wondered in from the garden where he had been sweeping off some leaves. ''You look, exhausted darling, why don't you put your feet up for a few minutes, I'll put this lot away.'' Maria began unpacking the shopping. ''It's okay, I'll get on with it.'' Sam always put the shopping away in the wrong place and anyway she wanted to have a snack in private. ''You finish up in the garden and we'll have dinner in half an hour, yeah?'' She said, trying to look cheerful. Sam ambled off, and she got on with putting food away in the cupboards. She opened a bag of chocolate raisins and popped a few in her mouth as she opened and closed cupboard doors and stocked up the fridge. She felt like she had to push on to get things done. She didn't have time to rest. It was easier to have a snack and carry on. The bag of raisins was soon empty, ''I'll just do myself a quick peanut butter sandwich to keep me going...''

Even though Maria had the opportunity to rest, her perfectionism drove her on. Her habitual way of dealing with fatigue was to eat high sugar and high-fat foods. She had established no other pattern of coping with the end of the day exhaustion and stress she felt. Her intense cravings overrode the offer of help. Maria needed to break this cycle.

For binge eaters, the evenings are often the most troublesome times. After dinner cravings for puddings, sweets or salty snacks can be overwhelming. Food is seen as a way to relax. Because of intense feelings of exhaustion, food is an easier option. It is less effort to sit on the sofa munching through bags of crisps or packets of biscuits than it would be to something more sustaining for body and soul. It's hard to break this habit. Everything just feels like too much of an effort. Brain fog and mental fatigue mean that cognitive pursuits such as reading, doing a crossword or learning a language is just too much effort. Even running a warm bath or doing some gentle stretches can just all seem too much.

It is important to improve sleep-quality for these reasons:

- To balance out hormones related to hunger and satiety.
- To lessen the intense craving for high-fat, high-sugar foods.
- Improved sleep will lessen the opportunities for night time binging.
- Better quality sleep will lessen feelings of anxiety, stress and depression which could all lead to a binge.
- Less fatigue will mean you will make better choices when shopping and cooking.
- You will be less tempted by fast food or takeaways.
- You will have the energy to enjoy more creative self-care activities or take part in sports or activities such as walking in the evenings and at weekends.
- You will enjoy quality time with family and friends. Sometimes even a phone call can seem too much when you feel exhausted.
- You will have the energy to get involved in creative pursuits such as painting, craft projects or DIY.

- Using your time more productively and creatively will lessen feelings of low self-esteem, boredom or depression.

The following are some tips to help improve sleep quality:

- Have a consistent bedtime and wake-up time, even at weekends.
- Avoid the temptation to catch up on sleep at the weekend and sleep in later.
- If you wake up at night read a book or magazine. Avoid screens because of the sleep-disrupting blue light.
- Eat well during the day and don't restrict food or skip meals.
- If you wake up at night, have a warm drink.
- Associate your bed with rest and relaxation. Don't work from bed or do work emails in bed.
- Set an alarm and get up early, no matter how tired you feel. Go to bed early that night to re-set your body clock.
- Modify morning behaviours: try to get outdoors for a walk or at least sit by a sunny window to eat breakfast.
- Avoid any late-night intense conversations or discussions.
- Use dim lighting in the evenings.
- Avoid intense exercise for two hours before bed–this can release stress hormones that will keep you awake.

- Avoid horror movies, thrillers, or disturbing news stories before bed.
- Practise mindfulness exercises such as journaling, meditation or a body scan before bed.
- Avoid eating lots of sweet foods or caffeine late at night.
- Eat foods high in polyphenols; these are contained in foods such as blueberries, strawberries and seeds.
- Prioritise sleep.

5. Mindfulness Practices To Improve Sleep Quality.

2014 research U.S universities concluded:

Mindfulness meditation appears to be a viable treatment option for adults with chronic insomnia and could provide an alternative to traditional treatments for insomnia. (1).

Compassion, patience, acceptance and non-striving.

By now you will be bringing these attitudes into your day-to-day life. If you need to refresh your memory, you can turn back to Week 3 when we look at each of these attitudes in some detail. Compassion is a key attitude to help you overcome binge eating, so I hope you are treating yourself with gentleness and care. Bringing kinder, gentler attitudes of patience and acceptance to daily life will help lower stress hormones and break the stress response. Practising compassion releases feel-good hormones such as oxytocin which helps to stimulate the parasympathetic nervous system, helping us to feel calmer. When our baseline levels of anxiety or stress are low, we will settle to sleep easily and wake up feeling refreshed. Accepting things as they are for today will help avoid the angst that goes with resisting or going against the tide. We can still make plans to change a circumstance we are unhappy with, but once the plan is made and we do what we can do to activate it, we can let go and improve our mood and sleep.

Resourcing activities/self-care.

I hope that you are establishing some habits of regular self-care. Self-care can be practical things, like sorting out your finances or tidying your desk. By taking actions such as these, we are easing the background nagging worry that goes with unpaid bills or a messy work environment. This, in turn, helps us to stay calm and sleep better. Self-care activities such as a warm bath or an aromatherapy massage will help soothe you and support excellent quality sleep.

Mindful movement. Gentle movement such as yoga or stretching is perfect for later in the day. These types of movements will ease out any aches or stiffness from the day, stimulate the parasympathetic nervous system and help you settle into a refreshing sleep easily.

Meditation. I have designed the guided meditations that accompany this book, to be relaxing and restful. By listening to them regularly you will be forming new habits to help you remain calm and centred. You may listen to them before bed, which will be effective in helping you to settle down to sleep.

You may sit quietly with your thoughts. In Week 1, I referred to this type of meditation, which can be a challenge for someone new to meditation. Remember, you are not trying to empty your mind; you will observe what comes into your mind, but not attach any emotion to it. When you are aware of thoughts, this is mindfulness. Sitting in silence can be calming and refreshing, but if you find you get into a struggle with your thoughts, then focus on the guided meditations.

Letting go. Letting go is a continuous process. It might involve letting go of minor things or letting go of more momentous events or experiences in life. In day-to-day life, we encounter many situations that can irritate or be upsetting to a greater or lesser extent. Don't let an upsetting incident or irritating person 'live rent-free' in your head. As best you can let it go. We might be bothered by disturbing memories or flashbacks. If you have some trauma that is disturbing your sleep quality it is important to get professional help.

Be present. By being present we are in the 'being mode'. We are fully experiencing what is going on in the here and now. This 'being mode' is a better state to be in to process any issues that have an element of emotion attached to them. The 'doing mode' is more effective for logical, practical issues when you are in a position to take action. For example, if you are trying to sleep and are worried about a job interview, being in the 'doing mode' is not helpful. Your mind will race ahead trying to project what will happen or presenting mental movies of the dire consequences of not getting the job. By considering the interview in the 'being mode' you can look at it in a manner that is more accepting of the various outcomes without having the urge to do something about it here and now. Once you have made the preparations, it is counter-productive to be lying awake at 3 am worrying that you will be too tired to perform well in the interview the next day.

Get out of the doing mode and into the being mode. By being focused on what you are experiencing in that moment, you are in the being mode.

Breathing. Breathing well, in through the nose, into the abdomen, slowly will lower the heart rate and induce feelings of calm and relaxation. By observing your breathing at regular points during the day, you will establish a habit of breathing well and maintaining a calm state. This means you will be less ruffled by the stresses of the day. It will take less effort to wind down in the evening and you will approach bedtime with optimum chances of a good night's sleep.

If you wake up in the night keep your focus on the breath. Practise just observing your thoughts; as if they were on a movie screen inside your head. Don't engage with them, watch them come and go.

Body scan. By now, the body scan will have become part of your daily mindfulness practice. You will have experienced how these quick scans can help you pinpoint areas of tension. You can then take some effective action, such as stretching or moving. This helps avoid the accumulation of tension which can keep you awake at night or interfere with settling down to sleep. If you wake up during the night, try practising a body scan in your mind, mentally focussing on one area of the body at a time and just observing what is going on. This can help direct your thoughts away from anything troubling you and help you drift off back to sleep.

Progressive muscle relaxation. This is a method of scanning the body but in addition to observing sensations, you will isolate your focus on one set of muscles and tense them up then relax and let go, moving onto the next set of muscles and repeating this action. For example, you might start with your left foot, focus on the foot, squeeze it hard then let it go, then move up the leg to the calf, tense up the muscles in the calf and then relax. You will then bring your attention to the muscles in the left thigh, tense them up, then let them go. You can continue this as you move around the body, repeating the process if needed. This will relax the body and keep your mind off any disturbing thoughts.

Mindful Eating. By eating mindfully you will be more satisfied with your food and less likely to wake up in the night with cravings. By eating slowly and mindfully, you are re-educating your nervous system to calm down. You will also avoid the chances of being disturbed in the night by digestive issues, as you will chew your food thoroughly and eating in an unhurried manner.

6. Practical Tips

This week we have looked at the importance of relaxation, rest and quality sleep to help overcome problem eating. The mindfulness exercises and techniques we looked at yesterday are most effective when practised within a lifestyle that supports excellent sleep and relaxation. The following is a list of some helpful practical tips to ensure top quality sleep and a more relaxed lifestyle:

- Use the body scan technique to check-in with yourself at regular points during the day.
- Ask yourself small questions as you go through the day. For example, 'how am I feeling?', 'Am I thirsty?' 'Do I need a break?' 'Am I hungry?' 'What do I need right now to feel more comfortable?'
- Build in a routine of practising a relaxation technique such as yoga or Tai chi.
- Practice self-acceptance.
- Listen to the guided meditations.
- Practice progressive muscle relaxation. This is a process of going through each set of muscles and progressively tensing and relaxing them.
- Get out into nature as much as you can. Take a mindfulness walk through a park or the countryside and focus on what you hear, see, smell and feel as you move along slowly.
- Connect with others with compassion and presence.
- Practise mindful listening. Don't interrupt or think about what you will say next. Listen fully to the other person and then respond.

In your journal, make a note of a few ideas you will use to improve your habits of relaxation and rest. Prioritise sleep and deep relaxation. See this as an essential component of overcoming binge eating.

7. Summary

This week we have looked at how stress, anxiety and depression are often interwoven with issues involving food. Being mindful of stress, anxiety and depression can help to break free from the control that food seems to have over your life.

We have seen how sleep deprivation or poor sleep can lead to overeating. If you have fallen into habits that are not supporting quality sleep, do be compassionate with yourself but resolve to make some changes if needed. I hope this chapter has underlined for you the role that sleep and relaxation play in supporting you in establishing healthy habits around food.

By breaking the stress response cycle and feeling calmer in everyday life, you will feel less exhausted. Being calmer and feeling like you can take things more in your stride, means you will feel less stressed.

By practising compassion, patience and non-striving you will be less inclined to get overwrought by the everyday stresses that we all encounter. Lowering those stress hormones means you will feel calmer. You will also feel more satisfied with the food you eat and cravings will be reduced. When making choices about food, whether, at the supermarket or the lunch trolley at work, you will make choices informed by what your rational mind wants rather than be at the mercy of your cravings.

Today, go back over some suggested mindfulness practices or the practical tips to help improve sleep and relaxation. Reflect on your habits and make a note of any changes you would like to make. Just focus on two or three. You can always return to this chapter at a later date if you still have improvements to make.

Above all, make top quality sleep and enjoyable relaxation a priority in your life. It is not an indulgence. By improving your sleep and relaxation you will optimise your chances of success in overcoming issues with binging or overeating.

Week Eight

Moving Forward

If you are facing in the right direction all you need to do is keep walking. **Buddha.**

"**M**um!" Maria's youngest son, James, was calling her from the garage... He had been there looking for his football gloves. As Maria went through from the kitchen, she could see the look on James's face–a mixture of delight and confusion. As Maria got closer she saw the source of his bewildered surprise. Her 'stash': a box full of chocolate, crisps and cakes. "Are we having a party?" He asked innocently. Maria felt a sense of shame wash over her. She managed to smile at him and shrug, "Maybe!!" She pulled the box off him and turned away, feeling oddly irritated by his discovery. Putting the box on a higher shelf, Maria sighed. She knew that she needed to stop this...

Meditation on Moving Forward

Take a few moments to get settled into your chair or relax back on a mat or bed. Focus on generating a sense of comfort and ease. Be intentional in giving yourself these few moments to let go.

Take a breath in and as you breathe out allow your shoulders to drop, your jaw to slacken and your eyelids to drop closed. Just watch the breath without changing it. If thoughts intrude, look at them with a sense of detachment

---

and let them float off as you concentrate on my voice and your breath. Allow the feet and legs to let go of any tension. Be aware of a sense of heaviness in the feet, legs and seated area. Take a full breath into the abdomen and the chest and on the next breath out, allow the ribcage to relax. Let the arms and hands to relax.

Observe any thoughts that come to mind. Be aware of your emotions as you approach the end of this part of your mindfulness journey. Can you find a label for any emotions you are feeling? Note anything that comes up. If you feel neutral and have no powerful emotion, either way, accept this without judgement.

Take a few moments to enjoy a sense of accomplishment in coming this far. This has taken commitment and resilience. You can use these qualities in your onward journey, in your mindfulness practice and your relationship with food.

Bring to mind the analogy of a neglected garden. This garden is a representation of your life. You now appreciate the garden and to look after it. The garden will not suddenly look well-tended and beautiful. It will take time, patience and trust to continue to grow. You will need to apply the same patience and trust to your own life. You will continue to grow and establish a peaceful relationship with food if you continue with the commitment and effort you have shown yourself over the past eight weeks. Continue to tend to your needs. Trust that these efforts will produce the fruits of peace, harmony and balance.

The small daily actions build up over time to form habits and practices that can help or hinder your efforts. All you need to do as you move forward is focus on one day at a time. Attend to the small, daily choices you make. Ensure they are healthy and resourcing. Show yourself compassion and care each day. Commit to making the best decisions you can for yourself each day.

Take a few moments to reflect on this commitment to yourself....

When you are ready, take in a deeper breath, stretch, stand up slowly and continue with your day, moving forward in perfect balance and harmony.

If there is a practice or an aspect of eating, self-esteem or body image you feel you need a refresher on, please take some time today to turn back to the relevant section in this book.

The most important thing is that you use what you have learned in the book practically. There is little point in reading the book and closing it and forgetting about it. It is here as a resource for you. I hope that you will return to this book in the weeks and months to come, as you go forward... You will probably see and understand more with each reading, building on your understanding, practice and application of the principles in the book.

By purchasing this book and working through it, you are investing in your most precious resource–yourself. The effort you have made in working through this book will be worth it in terms of your emotional, physical and mental health.

I hope that you take the time to enjoy a sense of accomplishment in getting this far in the book.

1. Keep Going

Relapse back into binge eating happens. Certain factors make it more likely, for example, the older you were when you started or the length of time you suffered from binge eating. Keep going, if you binge again, focus on harm reduction and get back on track.

By living more mindfully, you can be more receptive to the warning signs of a binge, such as:

- Your self-esteem feels shaky and the inner critic is taking over.
- You feel stressed or particularly anxious.
- You restrict food or skip meals.
- You try to over-ride natural feelings of genuine hunger.
- You engage in punitive exercise regimes with the object of looking better.
- Your self-care activities move away from feeling good to looking good.

You now have the keys to attain peace with food: guided meditations, body scans, mindful awareness, attitudes and mindful eating. By using these keys you will be able to tune into your hunger, your emotions, and your needs. By actively slowing down, focusing on one thing at a time, and by being fully present in each moment, you will feel calmer and more in control.

By applying mindfulness attitudes such as compassion, acceptance, patience, and letting go you will respond to irritations, stressors, or challenges with more equanimity and calm. Life does not have to be such a struggle. The build-up of tension that could lead to a binge will lessen.

By establishing an eating pattern that is based on wholesome foods you will avoid blood sugar crashes and overwhelming cravings due to poor nutrition.

You might feel that your self-esteem is constantly bashed by images of thin, happy-looking people. This could be on social media, television, magazines, and newspapers. However, we can exert some control over:

- What we focus on and pay attention to.
- The language we use.
- The choices we make–we might feel like we have no choices, but we are always making choices.
- The attitudes we bring to a situation.
- The people we spend our free time with.
- The material we read, watch or listen to.
- Our level of acceptance or resistance to how things are.
- How we spend our free time–no matter how limited that might be.
- How we tend to our health–food, smoking, alcohol, etc.
- Whether we drift along aimlessly, on automatic pilot, or live with intention and focus.

Think about each of these areas and consider the choices you make. This is not about assigning blame but it is about taking control. Think about what you have control over. You have control over the material you read, the people you spend time with, how to use your free time, and the food and items you bring into your home.

If you consider the choices you make daily perhaps there are a few you could tweak to be more supportive to you?

Get into the habit of doing an informal body scan regularly at points during the day to check in with yourself, to build up a steady ongoing awareness of how you are feeling in your body.

When you sense tension or stress, feel your feet, get grounded, and slow down your breathing.

Pay attention to what you are doing and avoid multi-tasking, deliberately slow down your movements, speech, and breath.

2. Making a Plan to Keep Going

By having a plan, the chances of you overcoming your binge eating in the long-term are enhanced. It will not just be a vague aspiration, but you will have something solid to guide you to keep you on track. This is your plan, based on mindfulness principles. It has to be tailored to your life needs, wishes and aspirations. Above all, I hope having a plan can give you a sense of being supported and guided. It is not a straight-jacket and can be amended as you require.

The objectives of the plan are to:

- Eat well and often.

- Attend to self-care.
- Manage urges to binge.
- Build-in enjoyable movement.
- Manage emotions and self-esteem.
- Enlist support and connect with others.
- Avoid getting caught up in the diet trap.

Plan.

Make your plan with a sense of balance and self-compassion. Rather than focus on an outcome, pay attention to your behaviours that will support physical, emotional and mental health. Make a rough plan of your daily routine that includes time for mindfulness exercises, movement, time to shop and prepare nutritious meals and some self-care activities. Include social time or time with a support network or medical team who are helping you.

Take baby steps.

Often one slight change will provide the momentum to continue with other changes as you go forward. Do what will be easy for you and if you do more, look on it as a bonus. For example, you might plan a ten-minute walk before breakfast to help you feel better and improve sleep quality. When you get outside, you might enjoy it so much you walk for twenty minutes.

Get support.

If you have Binge Eating Disorder, you must get professional help. If you suffer from depression, please get support. That being said, everyone needs support in terms of family and friends who can help by listening, offering emotional support and being there for you. You might need to enlist the help of family members in your household to pitch in with chores to take the pressure off you if you are feeling stressed or overburdened.

Allow for possible setbacks.

Do not expect yourself to follow your plan perfectly. There will be days that are better than others. If you have a day when you binge or overeat compulsively, get back to the plan as soon as possible. Avoid black and white thinking. Often, people will have a binge and think they have 'blown it'. You can get back on track and pick up where you were. Look on any setbacks as opportunities to learn more about yourself. To help avoid binges, make a list of the ten things you could do instead of binging. Stick the list near the fridge to remind you in a moment of temptation. Look back at Week 1 and pick out strategies that have been helpful to you in avoiding a binge or reducing the impact of a binge. Be prepared for the possibility of being tempted to binge again. The urge will not magically disappear but you can deal with it.

Allow yourself to enjoy the food at a social gathering or special occasion. Slow down and pay attention to the food and your surroundings. You need not deny yourself. By eating socially and taking pleasure in the food and company, you will be less tempted to indulge secretly later.

Celebrate, enjoy the sense of accomplishment.

Plan the next step. Think about what you will do next to build on your success and keep the momentum going. Go easy and steady; remember 'consistency trumps intensity' – no need to push too hard.

With these points in mind, your plan to keep going will have these headings:

- Nutrition.
- Movement.
- Connection.
- Sleep and relaxation.
- Emotions and self-esteem.
- Dealing with stress.

Nutrition

Depending on your needs, you could commit to eating three balanced meals a day and two snacks. You may want to do a meal plan for the week, or take a more relaxed approach but always ensure that you have nutritious food at home. You could note how and when you will do your food shopping.

Movement

Plan what and how you will exercise. Remember to choose activities you enjoy. You could commit to a twenty-minute walk each day and a swim or bike ride a couple of times a week. Aim for movement that is easy to fit into your routine.

Connection.

Each week make sure you see friends and loved ones. Make plans for visits or activities together. Perhaps join a dance class or a running club – this way you are getting in some enjoyable movement too. If you attend support groups or meetings, keep up your attendance and when you are ready, take on some responsibility to keep up your accountability. Be mindful of people who drag you down or trigger feelings of low self-worth, limit contact with them.

Sleep and relaxation.

Avoid getting over-tired. Commit to an adequate amount of sleep every night. Try to keep this consistent across the week and at weekends. Every day, take at least thirty minutes to relax.

Emotions and self-esteem.

Practise emotional check-ins regularly every day. Use your journal to chart your emotions. Be mindful of how certain people, places or events impact on you emotionally. Share how you are feeling with people you trust. Practise gratitude, self-compassion and self-care. Be on the lookout for people-pleasing and say 'no', when you need to.

Dealing with stress.

Look at what causes you the most stress and either ask for help, eliminate or minimise the stressful activity or think about how best you can manage an unavoidable stressful situation. If you feel chronically stressed, get support with this. Look back at Week 7 for more ideas on handling stress.

Record the headings in your journal and write what you will do each week to meet your needs under each heading. This is your plan to keep you on track as you move forwards.

You can take stock once a month or so to see what needs to be tweaked. We will look at how you can take stock, tomorrow.

3. Taking Stock

Today, I will provide a summary of the key points to keep in mind as you evaluate where you are at. You can return to these principles at any time. Think about each point and consider if you have forgotten or have overlooked anything.

I will break the summary up into mind, body and emotions. As you will be aware by now, binge eating or problems with overeating involves the whole person.

Mind

- Practice gratitude every day, especially for your body.
- Focus on health and well-being. Avoid diet culture.
- Be aware of what you are exposed to in terms of magazines, email notifications, Facebook feeds. Cut out anything that triggers feelings of shame or inadequacy.
- Build up a resource of self-care activities you enjoy.
- Recognise your needs and learn ways to meet them promptly.
- Use your mind to learn, create and discover new things that are not associated with diet or appearance.
- Let go of resentments or negative feelings towards others or yourself.
- Ignore the inner critic.
- Build up some tolerance to mild discomfort and sit with it.
- Use your mind to plan to avoid triggers and maximise success in terms of moderate, healthy eating.

Body

- Eat when you are hungry.
- Eat for good health and satiety.
- Stop eating when you feel full.
- Practise mindful eating and enjoy your food.
- Practise body scans to tune into how your body is feeling.

- Move your body mindfully in a way you enjoy.
- Show gratitude and appreciation of your body by dressing in clothes that fit and having personal care routines that make you feel good.

Emotions.

- Get support.
- Avoid isolating yourself.
- Spend time with people who are positive and encouraging.
- Avoid people-pleasing.
- Accept your emotions and work through any troubling feelings with compassion.
- Find sustaining ways to deal with emotions other than eating.
- Connect with nature.
- Practise gratitude.

At any time you feel you are drifting back into old behaviours, have a look at these lists and take stock. These pointers could help pinpoint where you need to readjust to get back on track.

Do you remember I used the analogy of learning to ride a bicycle back in the introduction? When riding a bicycle, we have to steer, pay attention, and make minor adjustments to keep our balance and momentum to move forwards. You will need to do the same with your lifestyle and behaviours around eating. If you lose your balance or hit a road bump and fall off, take note of where the road bump is so you can avoid it next time and get back on plan.

4. Mindful Ways To Recover From A Binge.

As you go forward, it would be unrealistic to expect that you will never binge again.

Recovery from binge eating is more about reducing the frequency and intensity of binges. By practising mindfulness techniques and prioritising your health and well-being, the likelihood of a binge occurring is lessened, but it might happen.

If it happens, the following are some practical tips to help get you back on track:

- Silence the inner critic. Don't let it beat you up. It happened, let's move on.
- Be good to yourself. Be a friend to yourself and exercise self-compassion.
- Ditch feelings of shame.
- Investigate what happened. Why did you feel the urge to binge?

    Consider these possibilities:

    Hunger?
    Anger?
    Feeling lonely/sad/down/needing comfort?
    Feeling tired / overwhelmed?

Make adjustments to your routine to avoid repetition. Don't let it become a weekly occurrence. Identify your needs and take action to get them met.

- Get back to your normal routine as soon as possible.
- Ensure you are eating nourishing food regularly.
- Get some rest.
- Get out of the house; try to practise gratitude for what you experience outdoors.
- Listen to a guided meditation or sit watching the breath for a few moments.
- Sit with the discomfort and reflect on how a food binge will not meet your genuine needs.
- Pour out your feelings onto paper – write about the experience in your journal. You could use this as material to turn to when you are tempted to binge again.

Look back at Week 1, Day 3 for additional guidance on recovering from a binge.

Tomorrow we will look at a comprehensive plan to get you back on track if you do binge or feel strongly tempted to binge.

5. A 7-day Plan to Get Back on Track

You might use this plan if you have had a binge and want to get back on track.

You could also use this 7-day plan as a proactive approach in avoiding a binge.

If you have binged, please forgive yourself. You cannot get better by shaming yourself. Be compassionate with yourself. Turn to Week 1, Day 3 and re-read what to do if you have had a binge.

You might not have had a binge, but you can see the signs that show you are at risk of a binge. The following are some situations or mind-sets that could either trigger a binge or indicate that you are at risk of binging.

Signs/ Risks of an impending binge:

- Being tempted to hoard your usual binge foods.
- Isolating yourself from friends and family.
- Feeling stressed or very anxious.
- Feelings of low self-worth or self-loathing.
- Focusing on aspects of your body you dislike and feeling dissatisfied with your appearance, weight or size.
- Fantasising about binging.
- Intense worry about an upcoming celebration or event that is focused on food.
- Restricting your food intake or skipping meals.
- Pushing yourself to exercise vigorously just to change your appearance.
- Constantly comparing yourself to others or images in the media.
- Feeling upset by insensitive comments from someone, related to your weight or size.

- An upcoming visit with a relative who always has something to say about your appearance.
- An anniversary of bereavement or loss.

The first thing to do is to make your health and recovery a priority this week. Look at your schedule for the week and write or record on an electronic calendar when you will build in time for:

- Shopping and meal preparation.
- Plenty of time to eat meals mindfully.
- Self-care.
- Alone time to journal, listen to guided meditations or meditate.
- Attend to any medical issues; for example, visit your health care provider for a check-up or some treatment.
- Time with supportive friends, self-help or therapy group.
- Time for enjoyable movement activities such as walking, swimming or yoga.
- Time in nature.
- Getting rid of any diet foods, magazines or triggering social media content.

You could look back at Week 2, Day 6 for additional ideas to help get you back on track.

Each day this week do these three things:

- Listen to a guided meditation; choose any of the meditations that accompany this book, depending on your needs or desires.
- Choose one section to read from this book that appeals to you, again depending on your current issues or concerns. Keep compassion and gratitude at the forefront of your mind.
- Use your journal to schedule in supportive activities and record your feelings and progress.

If you commit to focusing on the above activities, you will minimise the chances of getting back into a pattern of binge-eating. If you feel that you are at risk of a binge, by committing to this plan for seven days, you will be less likely to be overwhelmed by temptation and it will help re-set your behaviours.

6. Summary

If you have read the entire book this far, I am truly honoured and humbled to guide you on the journey to better health and peace with food.

You have come a long way and I hope that you are reassured that you are not alone. Binge eating and compulsive overeating are common problems that people are often too ashamed to talk about openly. Please do not feel isolated and alone.

We have covered a lot in this book. You can use the book as a reference to return to as you need to. Remember, recovery from binge eating is not one straight upward line. There will be set-backs and slips. If you still binge but the binges are less frequent, less intense and you are eating nourishing foods, this is progress.

Going forwards, bear in mind the following guidance:

- **Resource**
  Nourish yourself with nutritious food, supportive friends and engaging activities.

- **Review**
  Mindfully observe your habits, reactions and choices regularly.

- **Re-adjust**
  Make any small tweaks as needed as you go along. For example, if you find yourself drifting to the ice-cream tub for the third night in a row, plan an enjoyable activity for the next evening – perhaps a girly night in with a bit of pampering or a trip out to the cinema.

- **Relax**
  Everyone overeats sometimes. You are following healthy guidelines now, not strict rules. The sky will not fall if you eat a cake. Enjoy it and move on.

True health and happiness are an inside job. By investing time and effort into a mindfulness practice you are building firm foundations for mental, physical and emotional health for years or decades to come.

Genuine contentment with yourself will only come with full acceptance, compassion and gratitude.

I wish you well on your onward journey.

7. You Are Where You Are

Here you are at Week 8. Well done on coming this far. Like any journey, there will have been wrong turns or delays. We are letting go of perfectionism and accepting where you are.

Today, take stock of where you are at with your mindfulness practice. How are you feeling about food, your body image, your self-esteem?

Have you been able to listen to the guided meditations or practise meditation in some form, even for just five minutes each day? Have you found journaling to be a helpful exercise? Are you remembering to stop and pause at points during the day too?

Remember you can return to this book, again and again, to help keep you on track. If you feel you are slipping back into old eating behaviours you can re-read the sections for this week or return to a section you feel you need help with, at any time. Use the book as a guide and reference when you need to. Success does not go up in one steady line. Complacency can trip us up but by living more mindfully, you have a better chance of seeing the warning signs in yourself.

Wherever you are, you are not alone. Look after yourself and although I have not met you, I send out warmest wishes from my heart to yours for your health and happiness.

I Need Your Help.

That brings us to the end of the main part of this book. But before you go on to read the bonus information in the appendices, I have a small favour to ask.

Can you take a moment to review this book on Amazon now? Reviews are so important. The more reviews I can get, the more likely it is that Amazon will promote my book, and I can help more people with eating issues.

All you have to do is go to the book's page on Amazon, scroll down and near the bottom of the page, you will see a button on the left which says "Leave a customer review". Click on that button, give it a star rating, add any comments you want other readers to see, and the job is done.

An easy way to find my book's page on Amazon is to enter the product code, which is B08BXY9YLL, in the search bar on any Amazon site.

Thank you so much for doing a review.

Appendix 1

How to Download the Audio Guided Meditations

To download the eight audios that accompany this book, please go to web page

www.subscribepage.com/mindfulnessaudio2.

There is a quick email registration, then you will be directed to the downloads page. You can either listen to your audios on the web or download them to a device to use at your leisure.

When you register, you will also receive an email from me with a confirmation of the link to your downloads, which might be handy for you to refer to later. By being registered, you will have access to any updates and free resources I send out in the future. I'm sure you will want these, but you can, of course, unsubscribe at any time if you wish.

Downloading tips:

If you cannot access the downloads or do not receive my email with the link, the most likely reasons are:

There was a typo in your email address. This is easily solved by going back and resubmitting your email address again.

Your email service has put my email in the wrong folder. Please check folders like 'junk' and 'spam'. If you use Gmail, it might be in the 'promotions' folder.

There is some sort of blocking software on your browser or device. Try using a different browser or different device.

Just in case you still have a technical problem accessing the downloads page using the method above, I have a backup system. You can also get access by sending a blank email to mindfulaudio@gmail.com. Your blank email will trigger an autoresponder that will immediately send you the access link.

Appendix 2

Mindful Movement

You can do these gentle movements anywhere with no special equipment. For the standing poses stand on an even surface and push trip hazards out of the way. You may wish to stand close to a wall for support if needed. Take extra care if you suffer from dizziness or blood pressure issues.

Mountain Pose

Stand upright and tall; imagine a string pulling the top of your head up towards the ceiling. Tuck in your tailbone slightly and feel that your pelvis is neither too far back nor too far forwards. Pull your tummy in and bring your shoulders back, opening up the chest. Arms are by your sides. Feet are together, with equal weight on each foot. Ground the feet into the floor. Be aware of the sense of any energy flowing through you. Spend a few moments breathing deeply and experiencing the sensations in your body.

Tree Pose

Standing tall as before, you may wish to move close to a wall to help support you. Bring your attention to one foot, ground it into the floor and feel the strength in that leg, gently shift your weight over to that side. Bring the other foot and lower leg across the front of the supporting leg, just at the ankle. Bring your arms out to your sides and focus on a sense of openness across the chest, breathe well. Imagine you are a sturdy tree. Visualise any powerful emotion as the wind blowing through your branches. Tune into your natural resilience and strength. Tap into this strength when assailed by powerful emotions or urges to binge. Stay with these thoughts for a few minutes. When you are ready, uncross your leg at the ankle and repeat on the opposite side. Give your entire body a shake and a shimmy.

Full Body Stretch

Standing tall, take a deep breath in, as you do so, lift both arms above your head and stretch up. If you are comfortable, keep your arms up, stretch up with one arm and push the foot on that side, down into the floor. Repeat on the other side. If you feel this is too much stretch up as described and on an out-breath bring both arms back down by your side. Let the breath settle and experience any sense of renewed energy you may feel.

Shoulder Release.

Standing tall, clasp both hands together behind the back, keeping the arms low. Take a breath in and gradually raise the arms behind the back, coming up with hands clasped. Stop when you feel a stretch in your shoulders. Feel the shoulder blades coming together. Breathe in deeply, on the out-breath, slowly lower the arms and enjoy a release in feelings of tension.

Hands to Heart

Standing tall, take a breath in and stretch the arms up above your head, bring the hands together at the palms into a prayer position. Lower your hands in front of your chest with the arms bent. With your hands at your heart, spend a few moments breathing well and experiencing whatever is going on for you in the moment. Perhaps have a sense of gratitude for your body and your ability to move freely.

To Aid Digestion

Kneel down and bring your bottom to your heels, legs tucked under you. If this is difficult, you could use a cushion to put under your bottom. Straighten the spine and bring the head up. With a straight spine, bring the head forward and gradually start to lower the head towards your knees. This is a tiny movement. Be careful not to come too far forwards. When you feel your sit bone start to come up slightly, stop there take a few moments to breathe here. On an in-breath, slowly bring the head back up. This movement releases gas and bloating and aids digestion.

Appendix 3

Resources

Books

The Woman's Retreat Book, Jennifer Louden, Harper San Francisco, 1997.

The Mindful Eating Workbook, Vincci Tsui, Althea Press, 2018.

Body Positive Power, Megan Jayne Crabbe, Vermillion, 2017.

Mindfulness, Mark Williams and Danny Penman, Little Brown Book Club, 2011.

Living Beautifully, Pema Chodron, Shambhala Publications, 2019.

The Miracle of Mindfulness, Thich Nhat Hanh, Ebury Publishing, 2008.

The Power of Now, Eckhart Tolle, Hodder and Stoughton, 2001.

Podcasts

The Dr Carolyn Coker Ross Show.

Heal Your Hunger Show.

Quit Dieting for Good.

Life. Unrestricted.

Appendix 4

References

Introduction.

    1. Dr Carolyn Coker Ross Show, episode 46, March 2020.

Week 1.

Day 1.

    1. D, Baker & N. Keramidas. 'The psychology of hunger. American Psychological Association. October 2013. Vol 44. No 9. Page 66.
    2. Secrets From The Eating Lab. Traci Mann. Harvard, 2015.

Day 2.

1. Overcoming Binge Eating. Dr C. Fairburn. The Guilford Press, July 2018.

Day 3.

    1. Presence—Bring Your Boldest Self to Your Biggest Challenge, Amy Cuddy. Orion, 2016.
    2. The Craving Mind, Judson Brewer, Yale University Press, 2018.

Day 5.

    1. Bernard M Duvivier et al. *Minimal Physical Activity (Standing and Walking) of Longer Duration Improves Insulin Action and Plasma Lipids More than Shorter Periods of Moderate to Vigorous Exercise (Cycling) in Sedentary Subjects When Energy Expenditure is Comparable.* Published 13th February 2013; plos. org

Week 2.

Day 1.

    <u>1.</u> Lisle, D, and Goldhammer, A. <u>The Pleasure Trap,</u> Healthy Living Publications, 2003.

Week 4.

Day 4.

    1. <u>In the Realm of Hungry Ghosts: Close Encounters with Addiction,</u> Gábor Máté, Knopf Canada, 2008.

Week 5.

Day 1.

    1. <u>Shades of Hope,</u> Tennie McCarty, Putnam Adult, 2012.

Week 7.

Day 2.

1. Abraham, S.F. & Beumont, P.J.V (1982) 'How patients describe bulimia and binge eating'. Psychological Medicine, 12 625 – 68.

Day 5.

1. Ong, J et al. "A Randomized Controlled Trial of Mindfulness Meditation for Chronic Insomnia". Sleep. 2014; 37 (9): 1553-1563. Published 1st Sep 2014.

Appendix 5

Warning Signs of BED and How to Help– a Note to Family and Friends

The following are signs your relative or friend might have Binge Eating Disorder:

- Hoarding extensive amounts of food.
- Being secretive about food.
- Refusing to eat with the family or in public.
- Enormous amounts of food wrappers in the bin.

You can help them by:

Including them in plans to go out or socialise. Even if they refuse, keep asking them and make them feel included.

Build their self-esteem. Compliment them on the personal qualities and attributes you appreciate about them.

Listen to them without judging or criticising.

Encourage them to seek help if you are concerned.

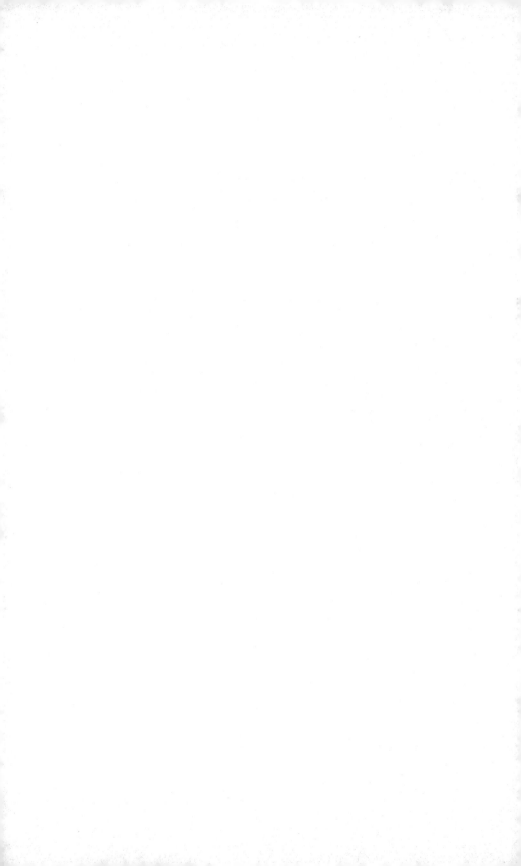

Printed in Great Britain
by Amazon

34161931R00148